Pain Truth Makes Sense:
Working Through Chronic
Pain After Trauma

Dr. Bahram Jam, PT and
Tashmeen Khimani Lalani, BA, RMT, Coach

Disclaimer: The authors and the publishers of this book do not dispense medical advice or prescribe the use of any treatment for medical ailments, and are not responsible for any adverse effects or consequences resulting from the use of the information in this book. Medical treatments, dietary changes or exercises should not be sought without consultation from a physician or a qualified health care professional.

Published by Black Pawn Press
Printed in the United States

Cover design by Justine Capiñanes

Print Version
ISBN – 978-1-949802-29-0

Table of Contents

The Pain Truth
An Easy-to-Understand Book About Pain
and What to Do About It

Dr. Bahram Jam
Registered Physiotherapist

To my wonderful parents,
My darling one-of-a-kind wife, and my
three daughters; Nadia, Tara & Roxana
who light up my life!
B.J.

Special Thanks

I am grateful for the assistance of the many people who have been invaluable putting this book together. My warmest gratitude goes to my colleagues and friends *Agnes Bellegris, Debbie Patterson, and Marla Perlmutar (aka the comma murderer!)*.

Preface

There are currently several textbooks and thousands of medical research studies on the topic of persistent pain. What is pain? Why do people feel it? Where exactly does it come from? What is the precise physiology behind pain? Most importantly, how can pain be eliminated or at least reduced?

The answers to these questions continuously evolve and change with each new research study published in journals around the world. Every year, hundreds of new studies attempt to answer these questions. This book's purpose is to provide a summary of the multitude of "pain" studies in ten simplified lessons. I make an assumption that most individuals who must cope with persistent pain do not have the time, energy or ability to research and comprehend this tremendously complex topic. The intention of this book is to take advanced scientific knowledge and present them in easy-to-follow lay terms.

Before going any further, two internationally renowned pioneers of pain education *Lorimer Mosely* and *David Butler* must be fully credited for their work in this area. These world-renowned Australian physiotherapists have educated thousands of health care providers on the topic of persistent pain. Their two books *Explain Pain* and *Painful Yarns* are a must-read for those individuals who wish to delve further into understanding and managing pain.

The sole purpose of this book is to help those who deal with persistent and medically "unexplained pain," to feel in control and optimistic about once again regaining their quality of life. So here is *The Pain Truth...and Nothing But!*

Sincerely, Dr. Bahram Jam, PT

Lesson #1: Pain is Good!

(At least most of the time!)

Pain is most often a good thing as it is essential for life and survival …without pain the body would not be protected and warned of potential danger.

Pain also helps protect the body until healing is complete or satisfactory; e.g. limping after an ankle sprain or fracture.

Pain, muscle spasms, muscle tension, muscle weakness are all valuable protective systems.

Pain is a warning signal that tells the brain to take action and do something.

Think of it as a home burglar-alarm system that warns us of an unwanted intruder. Pain warns the body of potential or actual danger …similar to a home alarm system.

All tissues have a pain threshold and a damage threshold. The tissue pain threshold should, of course, be lower than the tissue damage threshold; i.e. ideally pain should be felt before damage actually occurs …it would be silly if it weren't that way!

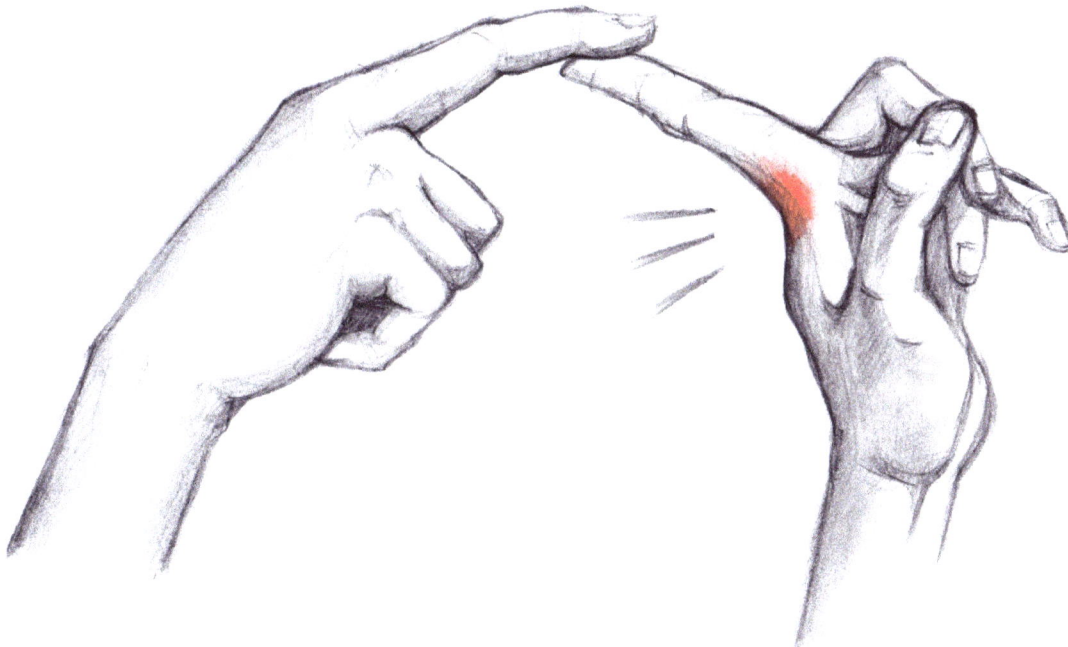

Bend your finger back until it hurts. Notice that pain warns the body of threat, **before** tissue damage occurs …once again, pain is good!

Look at the graph below and notice the double-sided arrow indicating the distance between <u>Tissue Damage Threshold</u> line and the <u>Normal Pain Threshold</u> line. Most activities performed throughout the day should be way below these two lines.

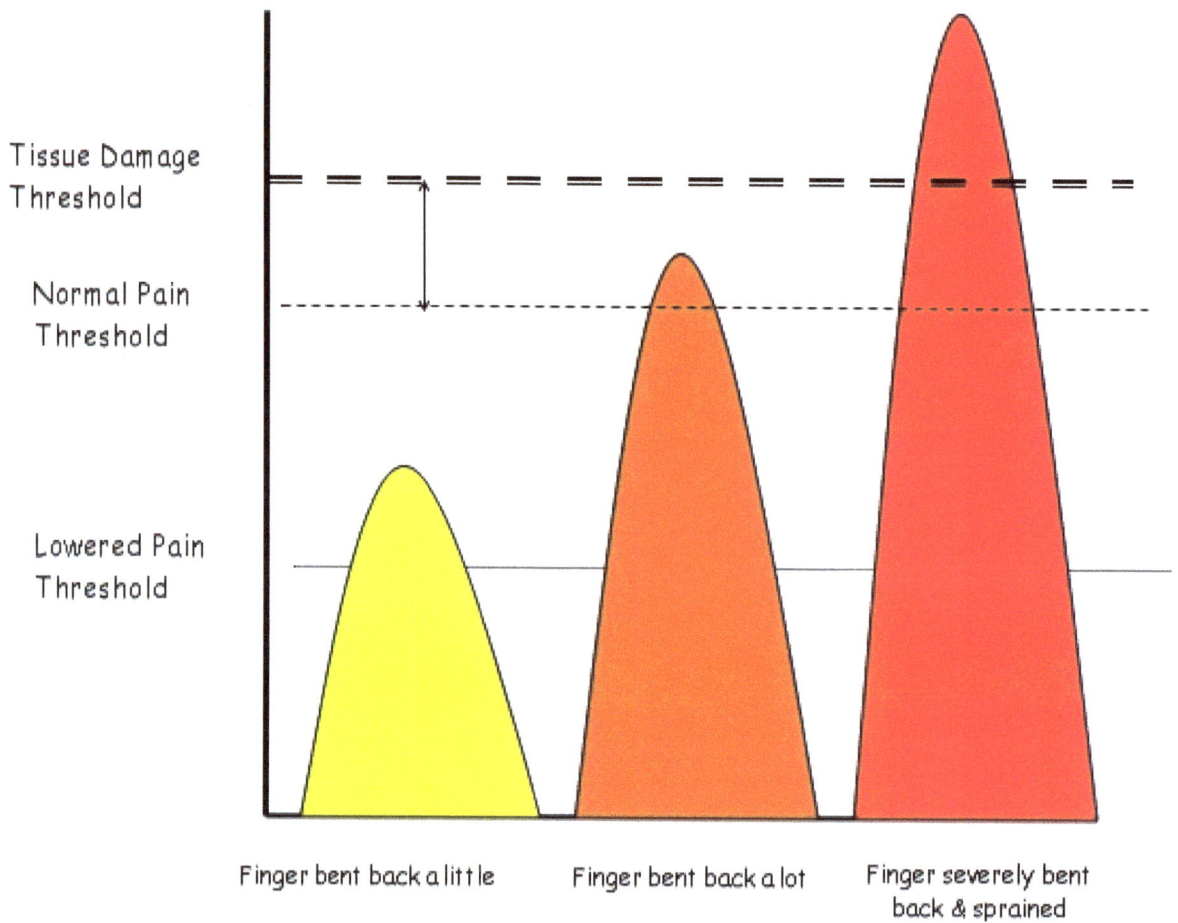

Tissue Damage
Threshold

Normal Pain
Threshold

Lowered Pain
Threshold

Finger bent back a little   Finger bent back a lot   Finger severely bent
back & sprained

Lesson #2: Why Does Pain Persist?

First, a thorough medical examination by a physician must be performed to rule out serious medical conditions such as rheumatoid arthritis, spinal cord injuries, infections, thyroid issues, possible medication side effects, etc.

Second, a comprehensive medical examination must also rule out less serious, but still medically important conditions such as fractures, torn ligaments, ruptured tendons, torn muscles, nerve root compression, etc.

The body amazingly heals itself in a few weeks or sometimes a few months. Normally as the healing proceeds, the pain related to the injured tissues naturally decreases.

A short course of physical therapy treatments including home exercises, mobilizations, manipulations, stretching, muscle retraining and postural education can often help speed up recovery.

Sometimes even after a course of good therapy and long after tissues have healed, pain persists.

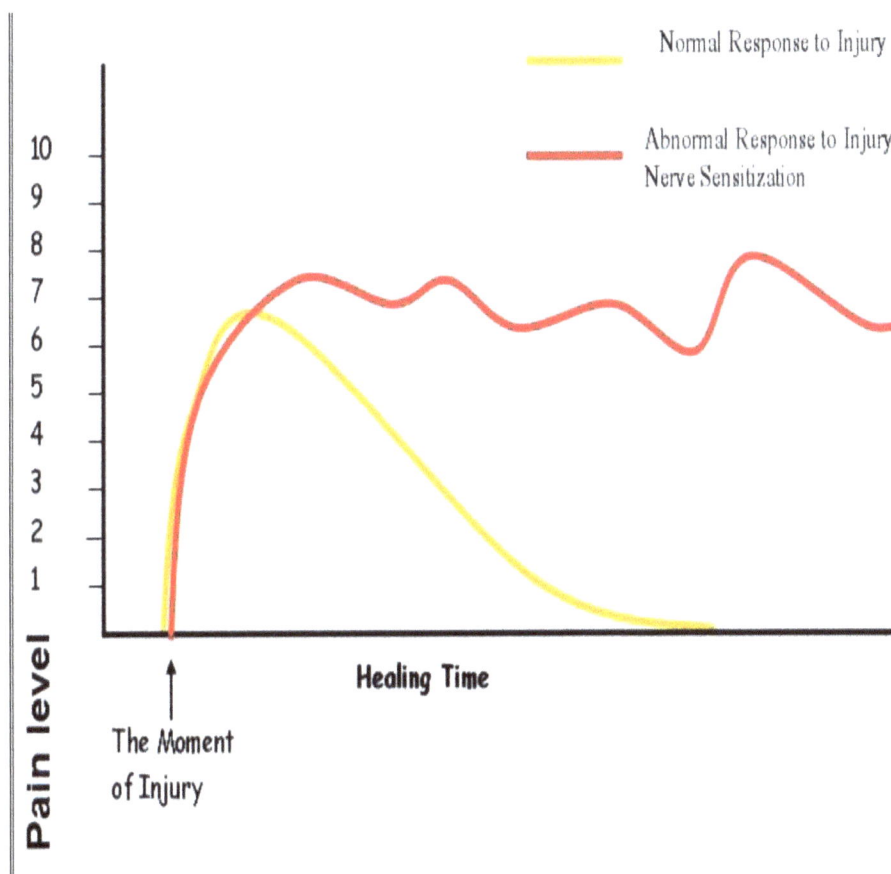

Question: What could be causing this pain if the tissues have supposedly healed?
Answer: A Sensitized Nervous System!

Burn victims suffer from severe pain long after the skin and the tissues have healed.

Their nervous system and their skin remain extremely sensitized even six months after the injury, when healing is actually complete.

Light touch or just blowing the skin on the back of the hand will produce unbearable pain.

Question: Will blowing or lightly touching the hand actually damage the skin or the tissue?
Answer: No, but the brain perceives that it may!

Question: Is the pain real, even though it has been over six months since the original injury?
Answer: YES! Absolutely 100% real ...ALL PAIN IS REAL!

Case Study

Helping Jane with Severe Hypersensitivity

Jane suffered a severe burn on the back of her left hand. It took many months before the skin finally healed. Coping with the pain required Jane to take quite a bit of prescribed pain medication.

Fortunately in time, Jane's pain decreased and was no longer constant. However, one year passed and Jane was still unable to hold a cup of coffee with her left hand without feeling severe pain. Any light movement, light touch or even gently blowing the skin on the back of her hand caused pain.

Jane knew that gently touching her skin was not causing any damage, but nonetheless, it was very painful. She was constantly fearful of something or someone accidentally hitting her hand.

Physical Therapy Advice to Jane:

Rub the skin on the back of the hand lightly once per hour. The next day lightly rub the skin twice in the hour. The next day, lightly rub the skin three times within the hour and so on. Also place the whole hand in a bowl filled with soft white flour and wiggle fingers for one minute.

Gradually increase the time the hand is in the flour each day for a week.

The following week, replace the white flour with rice. Another week later replace the rice with small lentils. The following week replace the lentils with kidney beans. Although it took several months, Jane did get the use of her left hand back.

What can be learned from Jane's situation?

Gradual stimulation is the only way of desensitizing hypersensitive nerves. This is a slow but sure way of returning to normal function. Without this gradual process, it is unlikely that Jane would wake up one morning and suddenly be able to use her hand.

Lesson #3: The Threat Value of Pain

It is the brain that always decides if pain messages are important or not that important.

Each person's brain is different and therefore every brain judges very similar situations differently. For example, visualize two people on a roller coaster, one person is excited and feels fantastic, the other individual is horrified and feels awful.

Why? Two different brains, two different perceptions! The brain constantly interprets all pain and evaluates its potential danger based on beliefs, memories and past experiences. If the brain believes it is in danger, it magnifies pain like a megaphone.

If the brain receives pain messages but it does not feel threatened or it does not feel it is in real danger, it muffles or even silences the pain. Basically, the brain feels pain, based on its potential "threat value." Research has shown that once people understand how the pain system, the nerves, the spinal cord and the brain work, it lessens the threat value and improves their overall quality of life.

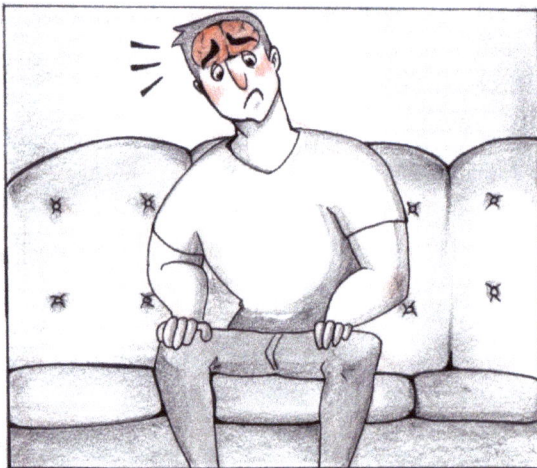

I have pain. It is dangerous…and there is nothing I can do about it!

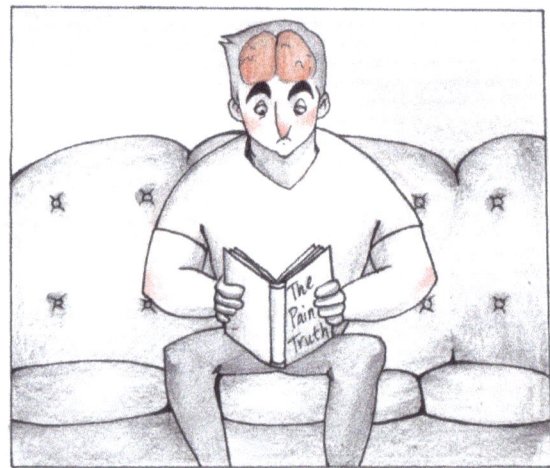

Reading The Pain Truth is changing the way I fear and worry about pain! I see light in the future.

Lesson #4: Is the Pain All in my Head?

Once people learn about this pain stuff, they sometimes become defensive and say *"So you believe that the pain is all in my head?"*.

The answer is "Yes, since the brain is in your head, and all pain is in the end interpreted in the brain, so it is technically in your head!".

The next question is *"Do you think that my pain is real?"*

The answer is **"Of course it is real, all pain is real,** but the source of some persistent pain is sometimes not from damaged muscles, bones or joints, but a sensitized nervous system.".

Although hard to believe, studies have shown that some patients just have to **think** about moving a body part and they will feel pain and witness actual swelling in the painful area.[4]

Even just thoughts and fears of pain can increase pain sensation.[5]

Simply thinking, *"If I do ……………………… (fill in with an activity), I know I am going to flare up my disc, my arthritis, my muscle spasms and my pinched nerve"* is a self-fulfilling prophecy.

Are you sure that just thoughts and fears of pain can increase my pain sensation? Yes, there are many studies to support that!

But don't forget, weak muscles and/or stiff joints can also contribute to pain, so they must also be addressed.

Lesson #5: Emotions & Pain

Hundreds of research studies have shown that our emotions influence our pain perception and nerve sensitivity. Some emotions, thoughts and feelings literally lower the body's pain threshold.

In fact, long after healing has taken place, thoughts can maintain the nerve hypersensitivity.

Our thoughts, beliefs and emotions influence our physiology including our heart rate, blood pressure breathing rate, digestion, muscle tension and nervous system hypersensitivity.

Studies have shown that just the fear of pain or the fear of re-injury powerfully influences pain perception. Thoughts (e.g. recalling something that makes you angry, preparing for public speaking, worrying about finances) will increase blood pressure, raise heart rate, cause muscle tension …and may increase pain!

Unfortunately fear is often magnified by the information received from x-rays, MRI's, other health care professionals, family, friends and the internet.

Degenerative changes, bone spurs and mild to moderate disc bulges are NORMAL and common in most adults …they are not a sign of damage or injury, Studies show that most people with "bad" x-rays or MRIs have NO PAIN.

Some individuals become stuck in the vicious cycle of persistent pain. In studies, negative emotions release stress chemicals, which in turn increases nerve hypersensitivity.

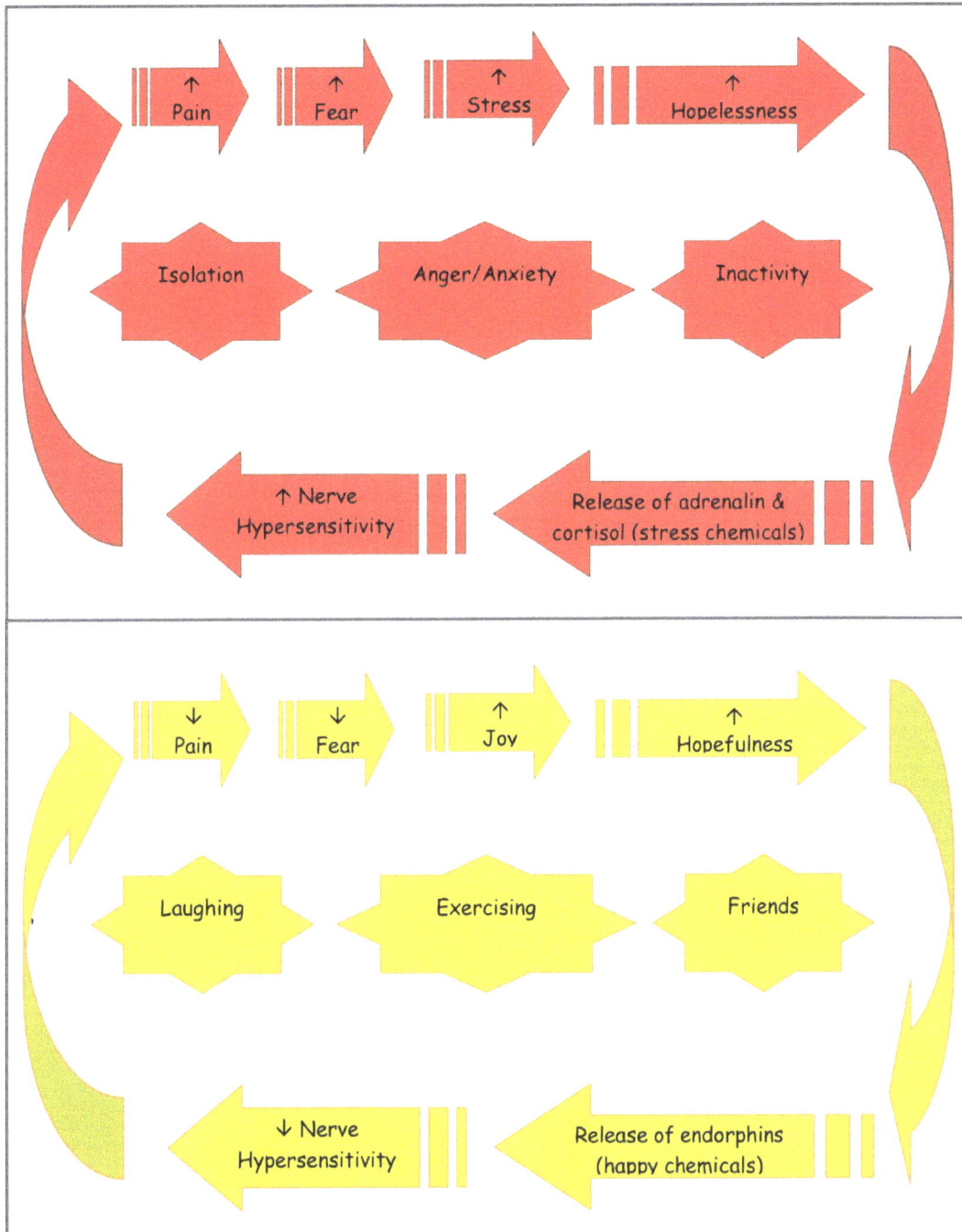

As you will recall, nerve hypersensitivity simply means that the normal pain threshold has dropped. Movements or activities that should normally not be painful are now perceived as pain.

Your Participation Section

Please grab a pen and paper and complete this "contract". Do not continue unless you do this!

I, _____ understand that degenerative changes, bone spurs, arthritis, and mild to moderate disc bulges are all NORMAL and common in most adults...they are not a sign of damage or injury.

I understand that studies show that most people with "bad" x-rays or MRIs have NO PAIN.

Signature: _____

Which of these 18 factors may be contributing to your pain?

- ❏ Fear of Pain
- ❏ Fear of Serious Condition
- ❏ Fear of Not Recovering
- ❏ Fear of Re-injury
- ❏ Worried X-ray Showing Arthritis
- ❏ Worried MRI Showing Disc Bulges
- ❏ Multiple Medications Ineffective
- ❏ Lack of a Specific Diagnosis
- ❏ Insurance Stress / Anger
- ❏ Sadness / Depression
- ❏ Hopelessness About Recovery
- ❏ Doing too much without pacing
- ❏ Withdrawn from Family / Joy
- ❏ Withdrawn from Hobbies / Sports
- ❏ Legal Battle Stress
- ❏ Family Stress / Anger
- ❏ Financial Stress / Worries
- ❏ Work Stress / Anger

Stress chemicals called **adrenalin and cortisol** are released during the "fight or flight" response, which help stimulate the nervous system ...they are crucial for survival.

These stress chemicals are designed to be released for brief periods during the ""fight or flight" response. Once the stress or situation is over, the body returns to its normal relatively relaxed state.

The purpose of the "fight or flight" response was originally to save a caveman from being attacked and killed by a sabertooth tiger. The stress always produced a **physical response** such as muscle contractions, running or fighting.

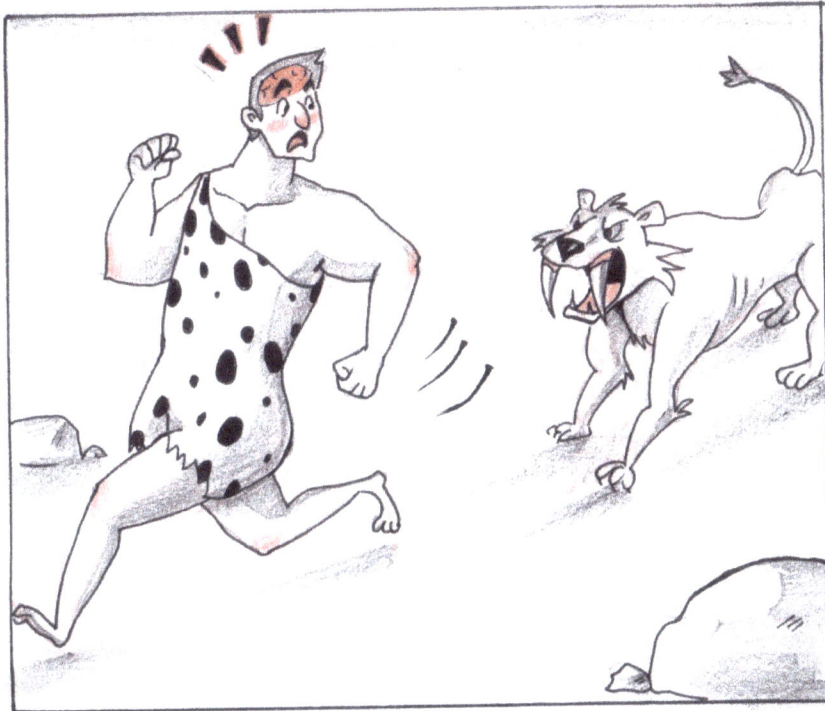

Although in the modern world we are no longer required to run away from sabertooth tigers, unfortunately, many people live in a state of continuous stress and anxiety as though they are constantly being chased and running for their life (metaphorically speaking!) in other words, they are in a chronic state of "fight or flight" and therefore release stress chemicals, **except now it is without doing anything physical.**

Notice the double-sided arrow in the graph below. It indicates the distance between the <u>Tissue Damaged Threshold</u> line and the <u>Lowered Pain Threshold</u> lines. Many activities performed throughout the day will be above the pain thresholds. The movements that were originally below the threshold are now above the pain threshold. The movements that did not previously hurt, now produce pain…Why?

This is called nerve hypersensitivity. The most important thing to learn from this is that the tissue damage threshold is significantly higher than the pain threshold.

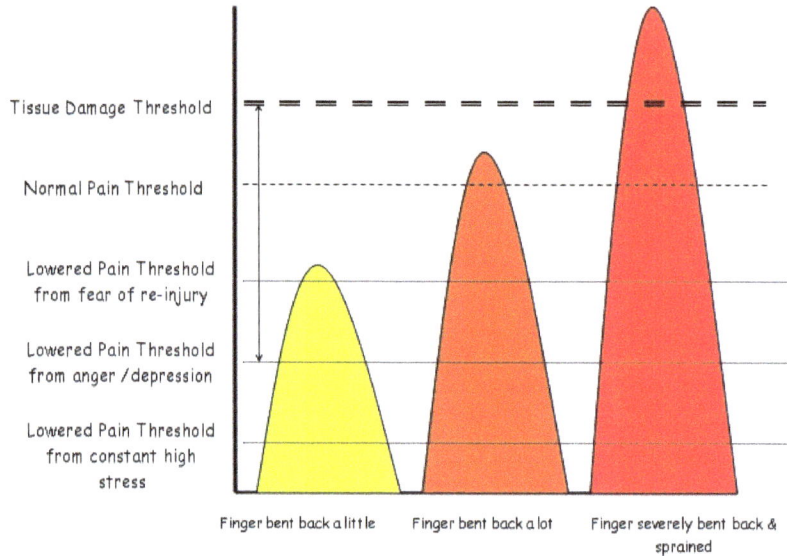

Tissue Damage Threshold	
Normal Pain Threshold	
Lowered Pain Threshold from fear of re-injury	
Lowered Pain Threshold from anger / depression	
Lowered Pain Threshold from constant high stress	

Finger bent back a little   Finger bent back a lot   Finger severely bent back & sprained

When someone has been a victim of a house burglary, it can leave him or her devastated, angry, fearful and, to say the least, upset. The door is broken, the house is trashed…it is an awful situation.

In the middle of the night, merely maintaining the thought that there is a burglar in your house would cause many physiological changes. Whether there is a real burglar or just the wind does not make a difference. Your brain is being cautious, warning you of potential danger, and wants you to take action.

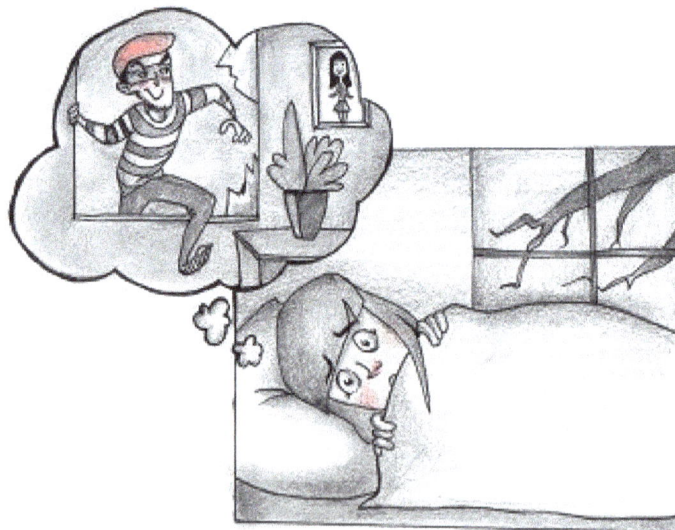

Case Study

Scarlet's Anger, Stress, Job, Boss, and PAIN!

Scarlet was a healthy 30-year-old divorced ICU nurse. She had been off work for the past 11 months due to severe low back and neck pain. She'd had months of medication, weeks of physiotherapy and massage therapy with little lasting benefit. She had had x-rays, a CT scan, bone scan and nerve conduction tests, all of which were normal. Instead of reassuring her, the normal tests actually frustrated Scarlet more. She was so desperately looking for a diagnosis and a cure!

She had seen a specialist who had diagnosed her with "arthritis" and "Fibromyalgia" (Translation: muscle fibre pain). Fibromyalgia is in fact not an accurate diagnosis, as it should more appropriately be called "Nervous System Sensitization" which can be compounded by life stresses.
Scarlet made attempts to return to work but it only exacerbated her pain, and her manager was not willing to place her on modified duties or change her department.

Desperate after 11 months of pain she visited me for a consult, here are her answers to some of the questions in a questionnaire:

How would you rate your current level of stress in your life?
Not stressed at all   Extremely stressed
0   1   2   3   4   5   6   7   8   9   (10)

How would you rate your current level of anger in your life?
Not stressed at all   Extremely stressed
0   1   2   3   4   5   6   7   8   (9)   10

How would you rate your current level of job satisfaction?
I hate my job   I absolutely love my job
0   (1)   2   3   4   5   6   7   8   9   10

Do you generally like / get along with your co-workers / your employer / boss?
I hate them   I absolutely love them
(0)   1   2   3   4   5   6   7   8   9   10

Please review her scores and see if you can figure out why Scarlet continued to have a sensitive nervous system. After more detailed questioning it was very clear that Scarlet still had:

i)   Un-resolved anger and stress from her divorce that was over two years ago
ii)   Hidden anxiety due to a history of emotional abuse
iii)   Extreme job dissatisfaction as an ICU nurse
iv)   Extreme anger towards her boss / manager who was unwilling to transfer her or modify her duties
v)   Financial stress due to her current unemployment

What can be learned from Scarlet's situation?

We all go through some degree of stress in our lives such as juggling between family and work. However, prolonged, ignored and suppressed serious emotional issues are contributing factors to nervous system sensitization.

Some authors have suggested that persistent severe pain may be a "protective" mechanism where we can simply focus and be distracted by physical pain instead of having to deal with EMOTIONAL pain.

Dr. John Sarno, MD has written quite a bit on this topic where he suggests, "Physical pain is designed to preoccupy the conscious thought in order to prevent the discovery of hidden and more painful EMOTIONAL issues in the conscious or subconscious mind."

While there is no question that your pain is REAL, but would you not expect your physical injury to have healed in a few weeks or months?

If you are currently under a lot of stress, it's possible that your emotions to some degree may be contributing to your pain. Sit down NOW and WRITE a list of all the emotional "issues" you can think of, decide once and for all to either deal with and resolve these yourself, or to seek professional counselling, Challenge yourself to find out if managing the stress in your life also helps you manage your pain.

If you are interested in learning more about this topic, read books by Dr. Sarno such as "The Mind-Body Prescription".

Lesson #6: The Outdated Pain Theory versus Phantom Limb Pain

Over 400 years ago, Rene Descartes, a French philosopher proposed a pain theory, which at the time made perfect sense. He suggested that when pain receptors are activated, pain impulses travel up to the nerve, up the spinal cord, into the brain and whamo …pain if felt! Similar to an electrical wire.

This simplified and outdated version of pain physiology, which some health care providers and patients still believe, is in fact untrue. Pain is much more complicated than this theory would have us once believe!

For example, 70% of all those who lose a part of their body feel sensations such as itching, burning and even severe pain in their no longer existent arm, leg, finger or breast. This is referred to as **phantom limb pain.**

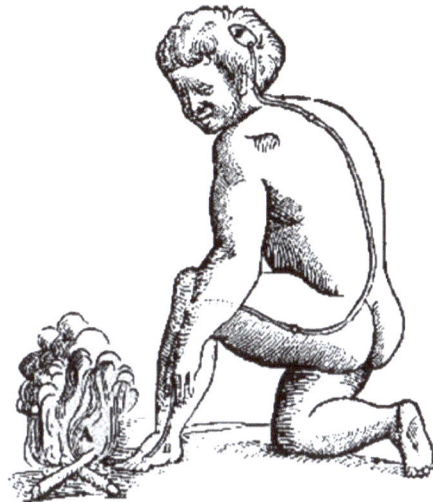

From René Descartes. L'homme de Rene Descartes. Paris: Charles Angot (1664)

This occurs because even without an actual hand for example, the brain has an image of the hand mapped out. The image in the brain is enough to produce pain! The body part image map that exists in the brain is called the Homunculus.

What you need to know is that the virtual body map in our brain (the Homunculus) can change based on usage, For instance, violinists and guitarists have a larger representation of their left hand, while the visually impaired that can read brail have a much greater representation of their fingertips in their Homunculus.

Our thoughts, the use, or lack of use of a body part **can actually change the Homunculus** in a positive or in a negative way.

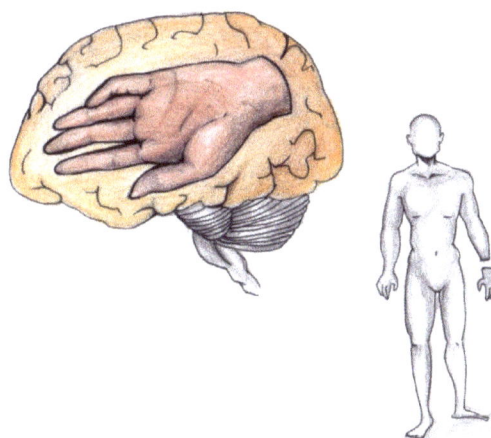

Case Study

A Fascinating Story of Abraham the Baker

Abraham worked as a baker in a bread factory. Due to a horrible accident, his right hand was crushed in a machine at work. The doctors had no option but to amputate his hand, Abraham went on permanent disability and did not return to his job at the bread factory.

One year after his accident, Abraham continued to feel some pain in his no longer existent right hand. The most confusing element in all of this was that he reported feeling okay on most days except for Sunday mornings.

Finally after much investigation, the problem was solved. Abraham's neighbor had the ritual of baking bread every Sunday morning. As it turns out, the smell of the fresh bread travelled into his house through his open window. The smell of the fresh baked bread was all that Abraham needed to trigger the event that occurred over a year ago.

To resolve this issue, Abraham was advised to close his windows on Sunday mornings! It worked. The pain ceased.

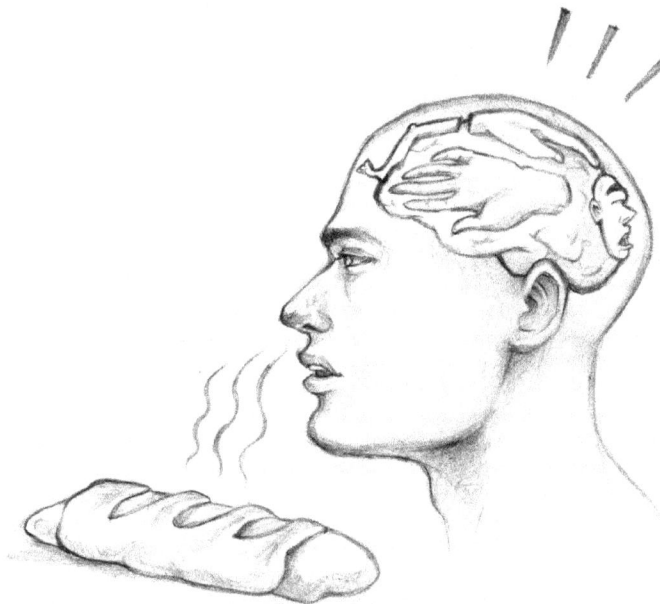

What can be learned from Abraham's situation?

If just the smell of freshly baked bread can produce REAL pain in a hand that is not even there, could other thoughts also trigger pain? What is your fresh-baked bread?

Could thoughts, memories, fears, and anger also trigger pain in joints and muscles that have already healed and are no longer damaged? The answer is in Lesson #8.

Your Participation Section

Please grab a pen and paper and complete this "contract". Do not continue unless you do!

I, _____ understand certain emotional stresses can contribute to my pain. The emotions may be (write the ones that you think may apply to you)

- ❑ Anger: *Briefly explain* _____
- ❑ Sadness: *Briefly explain* _____
- ❑ Guilt: *Briefly explain* _____
- ❑ Fear: *Briefly explain* _____

I also understand that learning to manage my emotions is essential for my recovery (e.g. writing solutions down for 15 minutes a day, mindfulness meditation, and cognitive behavioural therapy)

Signature: _____

Lesson #7: The Brain Does Not Want Us to Feel Pain …DPIS!

The amazing thing is that the brain does not wish for us to feel pain and tries hard to turn off pain messages; this is accomplished via the Descending Pain Inhibitory System (DPIS).

The DPIS is not a theory, it is real.

During religious ceremonies of self-mutilation, minimal pain is felt because the individuals involved believe they are doing it for a "higher" reason.

The majority of us have disc degeneration and disc herniations throughout our spine, yet most people perceive no significant low back or neck pain. Since the changes are slow, the brain has no reason to sound the pain alarm system.

Degeneration, arthritis, stenosis, disc bulges are not only common, but also a natural part of aging. The brain does not have any reason to sound the pain alarm system for wrinkling skin, greying hair or balding either (thank goodness, or I'd be in big trouble!).

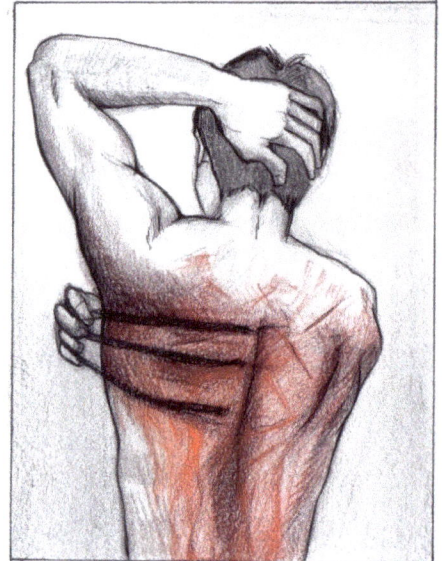

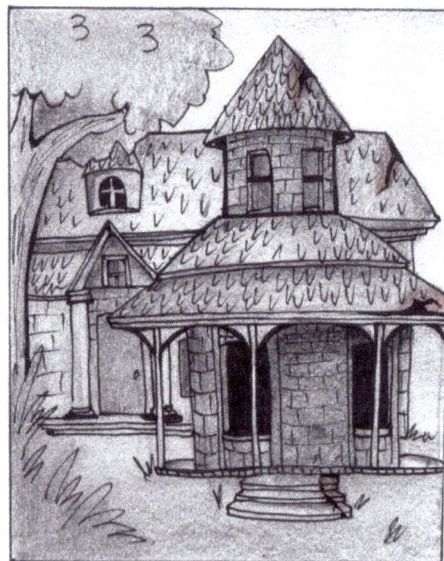

Think of it this way. Would your house burglar alarm system be activated if shingles on the roof were falling off, paint was getting old or the doors were becoming rusty and stairs becoming squeaky?

Lesson #8: What Does Nerve Sensitization Pain Feel Like and Why?

The classic characteristics of a sensitized nervous system:

- ✓ Pins and needles
- ✓ Burning pain
- ✓ Increased pain by small movements; e.g. slightly bending or turning
- ✓ Increased by sustained postures; e.g. sitting, lying
- ✓ Increased by no particular reason; e.g. the pain has a mind of its own, unpredictable zaps
- ✓ Trivial incidences cause flare-ups that last days; e.g. getting out of a car, walking in a mall
- ✓ The pain is increased by stress and anxiety
- ✓ The pain gradually spreads, even to the opposite side
- ✓ The pain may move around the body
- ✓ Pain even with rest
- ✓ Night pain

Nerve sensitization also means there can be actual physical changes in the spinal cord. There is enlargement of the pain pathways within the spinal cord that are normally small. In persistent pain states, the spinal cord literally amplifies pain or converts normal sensation of movement, touch or pressure to pain. Regrettably the brain now hears loud danger alarms coming from tissues that are no longer damaged or in danger.

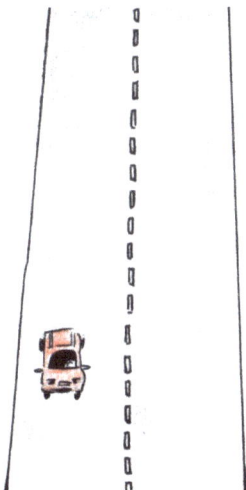

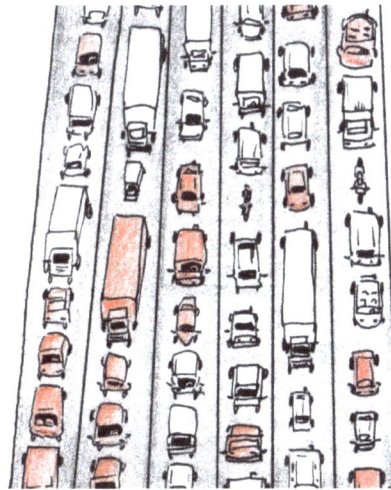

Changes in the spinal cord analogy: A single lane road gradually changes to a busy six-lane superhighway, which is not so good if the cars are filled with danger messages. In other words, the spinal cord is shouting into a megaphone talking to the brain.

As if the spinal cord screaming "danger" was not enough, the brain also goes through physiological changes. The brain itself becomes much more aware and sensitive in hearing the messages of pain, in persistent pain states actual changes in the Homunculus / virtual body map in the brain occur.

Pretend that your house has been broken into three times in the past month. In order to protect your home, you do the following two things:

1) Install a very sensitive alarm system with several extremely sensitive motion sensors that are activated by the lightest movement

2) Install really, really powerful and loud home sirens so they can be heard from several blocks away
This is all to protect our home and guarantee that it is not broken into again.

This seems like a brilliant plan, but there is one problem: The alarm system cannot be turned on or off at your convenience. It is on ALL THE TIME! This is very impractical, inconvenient and annoying to say the least. You would not be able to open your house door, open a window, and move in your living room without hearing loud sirens going off. Suddenly the alarm system that was supposed to help and protect you and your home from danger has become a nuisance and seriously limits life in your own house (aka body!).

All these physiological changes in the verves, the spinal cord and the brain occur to protect you in the best way possible. It is a great evolutionary means of survival. But sometimes these physiological changes outdo themselves and overprotect to the point of actually hindering the body.

Optical Illusions & Feeling Pain

Stare at the image below; are the horizontal lines straight?

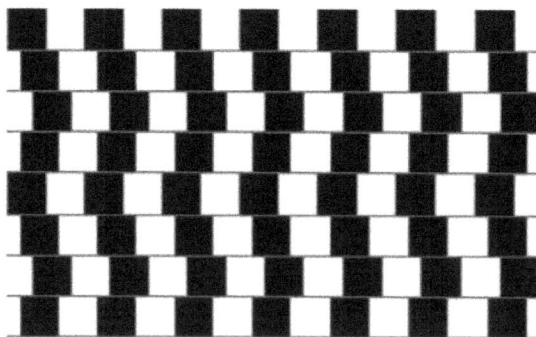

This is an example of how our brains can easily be fooled. The lines are definitely straight yet even though I have told you this; still your brain cannot help but perceive the lines as being crooked. This happens and is rationalized by the brain because of the **particular way** things are stacked on top of each other. **How is this related to feeling pain?**

Often our brain stacks up experiences and beliefs in a **particular way** and automatically perceives our body as being "damaged" (crooked) when in fact there is no "damage" as the tissues have healed (and are straight). If the brain believes the body is still injured and in danger, no matter how much you are told otherwise, the pain can persist. Here are some common examples of experiences and beliefs in those dealing with persistent pain.

- Internet searches increasing fear; so I must worry

- Multiple pain episodes; so it must be serious

- X-ray and / or MRI show changes; so something is damaged

- Pain is worse with movements; so I must be injured

- Been told of being "out of alignment"; so it must be true

- Belief that bad posture is the cause of pain; so it's my fault

- Been told of having poor muscles; so my body is weak

- Been told of having tight muscles; so it's my fault

- Many failed treatments; so it'll never get better

- Etc…

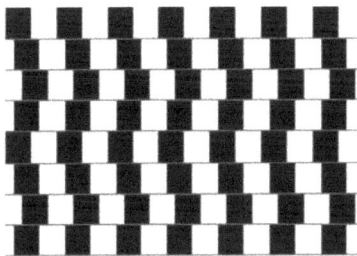

Because of the **particular way** life experiences and beliefs are stacked on top of each other, they contribute to feeling "crooked" and potentially pain. No matter how much a person is told the lines are straights, the brain can't help itself but see them as crooked, no matter how much a person is told that no structural injury can be found, their brain can't help itself but perceive that something must be injured. These ongoing thoughts and beliefs can lead to a sensitized nervous system.

Good news, the brain CAN BE TAUGHT to change and a sensitized nervous system can be made less sensitive…it just takes a new approach that involves the elimination of one inaccurate at a time. It will contribute to the "sensory illusion" and fuel a sense of danger and the pain experience, with the removal of many of the unnecessary beliefs and the reorganization, the lines will no longer be falsely perceived …and the "sensory illusion" ends!

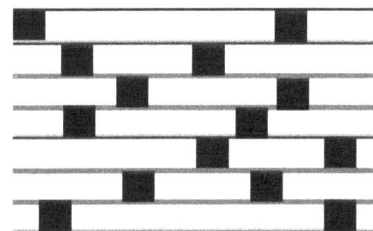

Child Falling off a Swing Analogy

I have frequently gone to playgrounds with my kids and have directly witnessed both of these fascinating scenarios.

Scenario #1: A child falls off a swing and scrapes his knees. He immediately looks up and makes eye contact with his mother sitting on the bench beside the playground. The mother smiles and gestures the child to get back on the swing. The scraped knee is forgotten, pain is put in the past. All is good!

Scenario #2: Another child falls off a swing and scrapes his knees. He immediately looks up at his mother sitting on the bench beside the playground. The mother panics, quickly jumps to the child's rescue, picks him up, the child begins to cry and will no longer go on the swing.

This time the boy's brain received signals that something bad had happened by falling off a swing, but more importantly the danger was confirmed by the mother's reaction. The caring and loving mother may have unintentionally prevented the child from getting back on the swing again.

What does this have to do with pain?

Sometimes we have an injury and we look to family members, health care providers, but worse of all, the internet to tell us how much "danger" we are in. Sometimes all it takes is a smiling person whom you trust to tell you that you can get back on the swing again, mot fear mongering web sites or health care providers.

Fear of Snakes Analogy

Some people are extremely fearful of snakes even though they have never even been bitten or harmed by a snake. Those who have extreme fear of snakes report of feeling muscles tension, anxiety, rapid breathing, and increased heart rate just at the thought of seeing a snake.

Some may have the same reaction with seeing a plastic snake, a picture of a snake or sometimes even with a piece of rope that may remotely resemble a snake. Now imagine if the person has actually been bitten by a snake before, then their reaction to a plastic snake or a piece of rope will be even more exaggerated.

Here are 3 important questions.

1. **Is the fear of the snake real?** Of course it is.

2. **Are the physiological responses such as increased heart rate, blood pressure, muscle tension and anxiety the person feels real?** Of course they are all real.

3. **Does it make sense for a brain to protect someone from danger by reacting to a plastic snake or a piece of rope?** No, but it surely happens to some people.

What does this have to do with pain?

If a person has had several episodes of neck or back pain then their brain and nervous system may become hypersensitive to even small movements and short periods of activities. Now slight movements that are surely not damaging can produce severe pain. Short bursts of activities such as gardening for 10 minutes or walking for 20 minutes that are not damaging can produce pain.

Is the pain real? Of course, all pain is real. However the pain may be a result of hypersensitive nervous system based on the brains past experiences and not related to injured tissues.

The judging brain: Are you in Danger or Safety?

From the moment you wake up and open your eyes, your brain is asking, "Am I in danger or am I safe?" Subconsciously, your brain asks itself millions of questions within the first few minutes of waking up and it goes something like this.

- *Am I breathing?* Yes? …good!
- *Can I move my arms and legs?* Yes? …good! I'll try getting out of bed.
- *Am I thirsty?* Yes? …better have something to drink after I get out of bed.
- *Do I have to go to the bathroom?* Yes? …better get out of bed now!
- *Is the bathroom floor cold?* Okay, I'll put on my slippers.

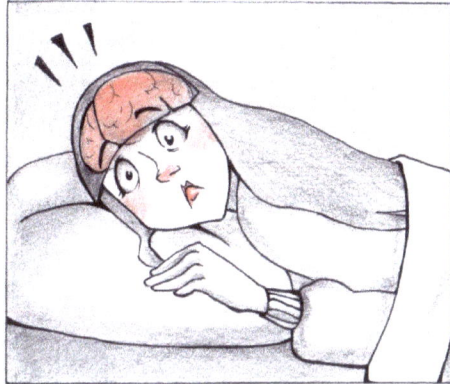

And so on and so forth …and for the entire day your brain will process billions of information to help keep you comfortable, safe and out of danger.

Imagine that your brain is holding an apothecary scale and is constantly judging if it is physically, psychologically and emotionally more in DANGER or in SAFETY. If the scale tips more towards the DANGER side, the nervous system becomes more sensitive to pain. If the scale tips more towards the SAFETY side, the nervous system remains relaxed and less sensitive to pain.

Which side of the scale will your brain judge to be more dominant? …the DANGER side or the SAFETY side? Since the nervous system is constantly judging if it is more emotionally and physically in DANGER or in SAFETY, if it perceived it is in DANGER, it becomes hypersensitive and focuses on experiencing pain in order to protect you.

If it perceived it is more in SAFETY, it remains calm and focuses on experiencing pleasurable activities.

Examples of Experiencing Danger	Examples of Experiencing Safety
Difficulty breathing/shortness of breath	Awareness that you can comfortably breathe
Worry and fear of X-Ray and MRI results	Awareness that "abnormalities" are common
Fear of going out of the house	Walking in the park/enjoying nature
Dealing with insurance companies	Mindfulness meditation
Staying alone at home	Hanging out with friends/family
Conflicting message from health care providers	Trusting a health care provider
Relying on passive treatments such as pills and machines	Relying on self. Feeling in control and in charge of your well-being

This list can go on and on. The point is if the brain perceives greater danger than safety, it will feel threatened and will do everything to protect itself, which includes produce pain.

Your simple goal must be to reduce the number and the intensity of danger factors and at the same time increase the number of and the intensity of safety factors that you experience on a daily basis.

Regretfully, a person who falls into the persistent pain cycle gets really good at focusing on their dangers and stops focusing on all the safeties in their life. Although the safety list may be a lot longer than the danger list, the brain naturally focuses on potential dangers for survival.

The only way focus on dangers can be reduced is to make continuous conscious efforts to shift your focus on the safeties. This is certainly not an easy task but it is definitely possible as the brain can change based on how we choose to think.

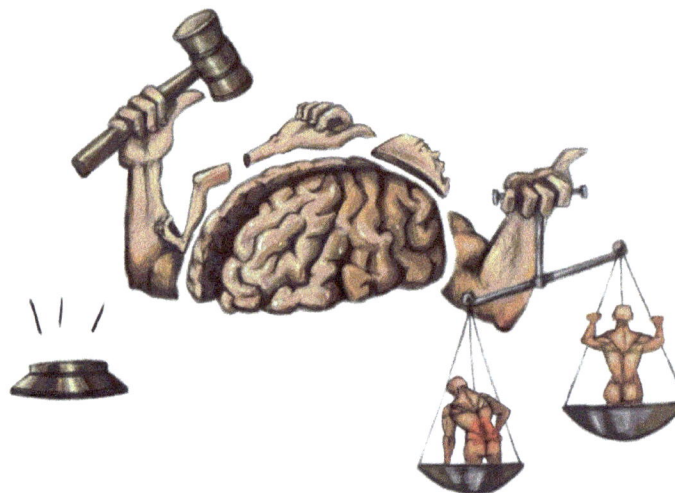

Please complete the SAFETY & DANGER questionnaire on www.ThePainTruth.org and write down your scores on a piece of paper.

If your DANGER score is higher than your SAFETY score, please consider completing the 6-12 week *Pain Truth program* with the assistance of a *Pain Truth Certified* (PTC) health care provider.

The aim of the program will be to MAXIMIZE your SAFETY score and MINIMIZE your DANGER score, which may result in you having a **less sensitive nervous system**.

If you are not yet sure about this program, that is perfectly okay. You may still visit www.ThePainTruth.org and click on The Pain Truth Program Videos and choose from any of the 10 SAFETY or 10 DANGER factors that you wish to learn about and potentially address by viewing the relevant videos in any of the sections.

You will learn from the videos that the pain experience is complex and that everyone is unique needing different factors in their life to be addressed. Perhaps some of the videos may partly explain YOUR ongoing pain experience and help you in your recovery, after all...

"The hardest pain to endure is an unexplained one."

The key to your recovery is returning to meaningful and enjoyable life activities.

The aim of the Pain Truth program is to assist you in determining what those life activities are. With guidance from your *Pain Truth Certified (PTC)* health care provider, you will set goals and detailed steps on how to achieve them.

Pain is an opinion of the brain and that opinion can be changed when the brain is provided with more accurate and positive information.

You must replace several of the inaccurate beliefs that you may currently have about your pain with more accurate and empowering ones. This will inevitably help reduce your sense of danger, increase your sense of safety and **reduce the sensitivity of your nervous system.**

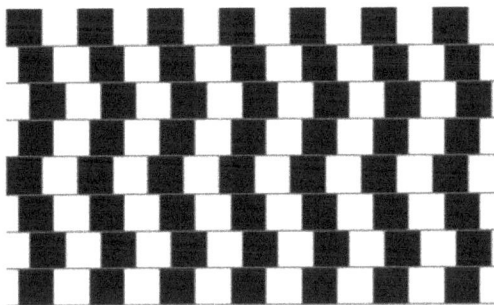

Perception that your body is "crooked" and injured.	Perception that your body is okay and resilient.

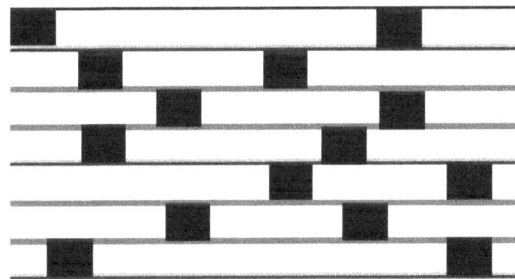

The Pain Truth program is NOT designed to eliminate pain, but to change your current understanding and your relationship with pain. If you are looking for a magic cure, then this program is currently not for you.

However, if you are looking for ways of improving the quality of your life by returning to some of the activities that you once enjoyed, then please consider viewing the introductory videos on www.ThePainTruth.org. All the content on this website is complimentary.

Write down a plan: The brain is amazing; it will not do anything unless it has a purpose. If it has a clear purpose and a goal it will do everything to achieve it.

Grab a piece of paper and write down what you would ideally like to be able to do in 3 months, one year and five years from now. Sorry, being pain-free cannot be a goal. Without clear and exciting goals, your brain will find it hard to get motivated to do anything including just getting out of bed.

Go ahead, write down on a piece of paper all the things that you would like to achieve in your career, physical health, and socially. Then break the goals down to smaller bits with a timeline to do them. **This is a key factor in your recovery.**

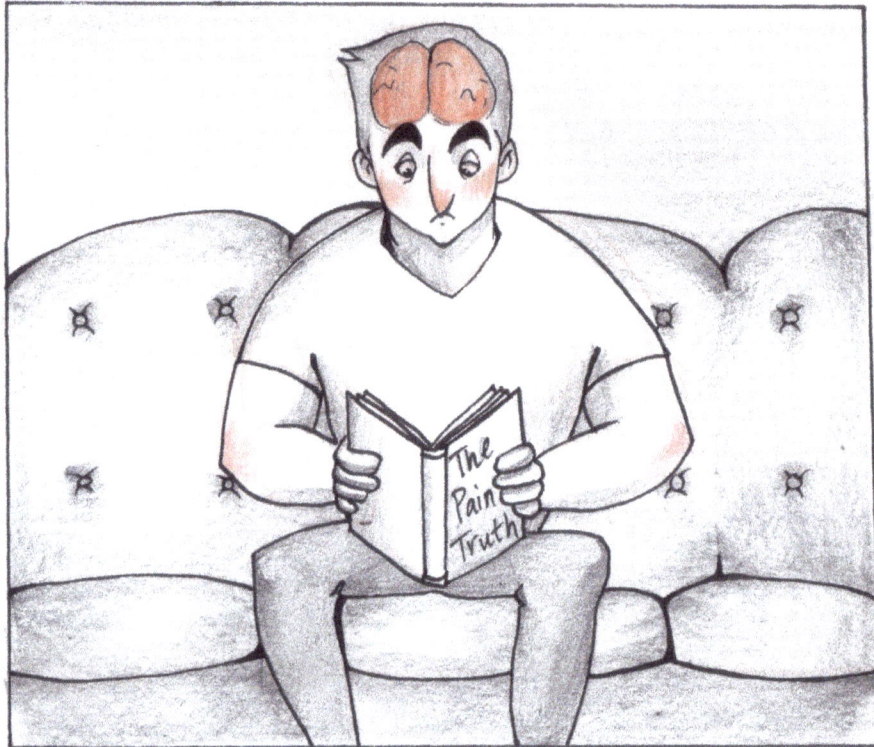

Lesson #9: What Can You Do About Pain?

Muscles become unhealthy and weak when they are underused. They thrive on movement and reasonable contraction.

Spinal discs are extremely strong but become unhealthy with prolonged inactivity, bed rest, or sitting. The discs thrive on movement and reasonable compression.

We all experience natural degeneration and wear and tear in our joints. But joints are much more likely to become unhealthy and painful when they are underused. Joints in our body also thrive on regular movement and reasonable compression.

What can you do? Immediately start a gentle but **progressive walking program, strength training program, flexibility program, Tai Chi, Yoga, aqua-fitness, cycling, and any specific exercises** recommended by your physical therapist.

In addition to being physically active, do not underestimate the value of relaxation, meditation and breathing, which will be discussed later.

Studies have shown that patients who learn to actively cope with, and not fear pain, have had better recovery than those who passively cope with pain.

Your Participation Section

Please grab a pen and paper and complete this "contract". Do not continue unless you do!

I, _____ understand and will do some form of an aerobic exercise program such as _____ EVERY DAY as I now realize it is a MUST for my recovery.

Signature: _____

Passive Coping Strategies

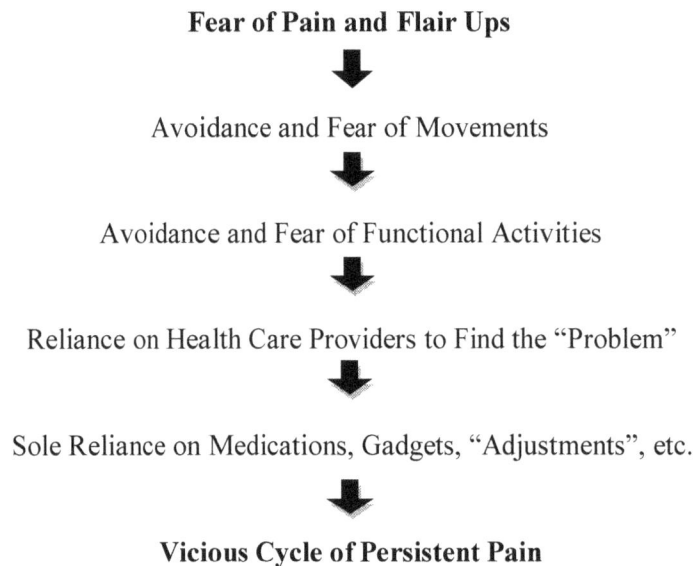

Fear of Pain and Flair Ups

⬇

Avoidance and Fear of Movements

⬇

Avoidance and Fear of Functional Activities

⬇

Reliance on Health Care Providers to Find the "Problem"

⬇

Sole Reliance on Medications, Gadgets, "Adjustments", etc.

⬇

Vicious Cycle of Persistent Pain

Active Coping Strategies

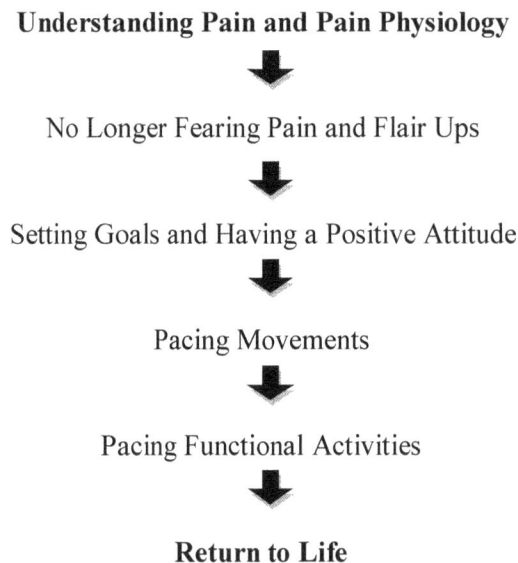

Understanding Pain and Pain Physiology

⬇

No Longer Fearing Pain and Flair Ups

⬇

Setting Goals and Having a Positive Attitude

⬇

Pacing Movements

⬇

Pacing Functional Activities

⬇

Return to Life

If you feel you require assistance in your goal setting in order to return to your 'normal life', I highly recommend that you consult a health care provider who is knowledgeable about pain science. A Pain Truth Certified health care provider can be found on www.ThePainTruth.org.

Case Study

Sam's Dependence on Medications and Passive Coping Skills

Sam had a fall and injured his back. After seeing the advertisements on the television, he took a few over-the-counter medications to relieve his pain. They did work and 'masked' his pain alarm system and reduced his protective muscle spasms. However, thinking that he was 'cured' as the alarm bells had been silenced, he painted his garage door. The next day, Sam had a lot of difficulty getting out of bed due to pain, stiffness and more muscle spasms.

He visited his family physician who prescribed 'stronger' medications. Although the new stronger medications did not completely silence the pain, they did help muffle the pain alarm bells. Assuming any activity would reinjure his back, Sam avoided most physical activities, exercises and household chores.

He believed that the medications would eventually completely eliminate his pain, and only then he would get back to physical activity. Unfortunately 6 months later, Sam still had back pain, which had spread over a larger area.

Every day Sam took a concoction of different addictive painkillers. Some of the pills that used to 'work' no longer helped him. Sadly he waited and waited, month after month for the pills, massage, tingling machines and regular spinal 'adjustments' to eventually 'cure' him.

What Can We Learn From Sam?

Firstly, in the acute stage of his injury Sam should have appreciated that pain was a "good thing". Pain was protecting him and giving him guidance of what he could and could not do.

Artificially shutting pain off with pills, then resuming all normal physical activities may not be wise after a recent injury. The body needs a few days or weeks to heal. Therefore, pain is a good guide to how much activity one can do in the early days after an injury.

Secondly, there are no medications or passive treatments that will ever replace gradual physical exercise and activity. Prolonged rest will inevitably weaken muscles, tendons, joints and discs. A weak body is far more prone to re-injury.

Waiting to be completely pain-free before resuming activity will often lead to 'chronic pain and disability'. Sam may have avoided the pain cycle if he had slowly paced himself back to activity, **even if he had some pain.**

The Three Possible Options and the Do's and Don'ts of Dealing with Persistent Pain

☒ **Option #1**: No Pain, No Gain

It is a bad idea to ignore your pain! This is because ignoring pain will likely end up causing you more pain in the long run. Acting like a martyr about the pain and pushing through it rarely works. Chances are you already know that by ignoring pain, you simply flare up. This causes your nerves to become even more sensitized in order to improve their warning capability!

Do Not Ignore Your Pain.

☒ **Option #2**: Always Listen to your Pain

Always listening to your pain is another bad idea! By intentionally avoiding activities, you will become a slave to the pain and constantly fear it. You may not even get out of bed, walk, sit, stand, lift, move or go to work. Resting and waiting for the pain to go away is okay after a recent injury, but harmful once tissues are healed.

Do Not Always Listen to Your Pain.

☑ **Option #3A**: Do Understand Pain and Do Not Fear Pain

Pain does not always mean that there is harm or damage occurring to tissues. Accept that persistent pain is often a result of physiological changes in the nerves, the spinal cord and the brain. It is sometimes the nervous system trying to intentionally magnify pain long after your tissues have healed. It does this in order to protect you.

☑ **Option #3B**: Do Slowly Pace Yourself Back to Activity

<u>Your Participation Section</u>

Please grab a pen and paper and complete this "contract". Do not continue unless you do!

I, _____ understand the negative cycle of passive coping strategies and fully understand the potential positive cycle of active coping strategies.

I also understand that reducing my fears about pain and gradually pacing myself back to physical activity / work are essential for my recovery.

Signature: _____

Easing into Activity Levels

First, find your "**easy activity**" level. What is the "easy activity" level? It is the level of physical activity that you are confident will not increase your pain. That could be three minutes of walking, or climbing five steps, or lifting arms overhead two times, washing four pieces of dishes, etc.

The secret to recovery is doing the "**easy activity**" as often as possible without flaring up. **Your nerves will gradually become less sensitive as they have nothing to fear.**

Gradually increase your "**easy activity**" by a very small amount. Walk for four minutes instead of three, wash five pieces of dishes instead of four. I hope that after all you have learned about pain threshold, you realize that even if walking for four minutes or washing five dishes produces some pain, you could certainly have not damaged anything in your body.

There is no doubt that in time, the nerves will simply become less sensitive and the Tissue Pain Threshold levels will go up again.

It is not recommended to "just ignore your pain," as it simply does not work. You need to appreciate that the pain exists, but that it is a false alarm.

Let's take for example that one of your goals is to be able to walk for one hour like you used to before you had pain. That seems unrealistic when for the past year, only 15 minutes of walking has caused you a lot of pain.

Step #1: Let's assume your "**easy activity**" is walking for three minutes. You are quite confident that if you simply walked either on a treadmill or outdoors for just three minutes, it would not cause you to flare up …excellent.

Step #2: Then set the goal of increasing your walking by ONLY a minute. You can be confident that just an extra minute could not possibly damage or harm any tissue. Even if you feel that you can walk for at least another ten minutes, DO NOT do it!

Step #3: Increase your walking until you get to your one hour of walking goal within two months. A goal that seemed so unachievable is now realistic.

Sample Progressive Program

Day 1	Walk 3 minutes ("easy activity")
Day 2	Walk 3 minutes and climb up and down 2 steps
Day 3	Walk 4 minutes and climb up & down 3 steps
Day 4	Walk 5 minutes and climb up & down 4 steps
Day 5	Walk 5 minutes and climb up & down 5 steps

Day 30   Walk 30 minutes and climb up & down 30 steps

Day 60   Walk 60 minutes and climb up & down 60 steps

Too often individuals who are coping with persistent pain simply dive into an activity, overdo it, and flare up. The secret to continuous improvement without flare-ups is taking small, gradual baby steps.

Pushing hard beyond the pain barrier is often a guarantee for flare-ups. It is not a wise idea to try a five-kilometre jog, play a full game of tennis, or do three hours of gardening if you have not been training for many weeks.

Just like in the story of the tortoise and the rabbit – slow and steady wins the race!

Your Participation Section

Please grab a pen and paper and complete this "contract". Do not continue unless you do this!

I, _____ understand the concept of "easy activity" that I must do EVERY DAY. My three "easy activities" include:

1)
2)
3)

(e.g. Walk on treadmill for five minutes. Clean the house for 10 minutes. Lift a 2Kg box 10 times. Light gardening for 15 minutes. Golfing five holes.)

Signature: _____

Too often individuals who are coping with persistent pain simply dive into an activity, overdo it, fatigue and flare up. The secret to achieving any health goal is to take small, gradual baby steps. Pacing ensures that the goal will be reached, and in time the nerves will simply become less sensitive.

Your Participation Section

Please grab a pen and paper and complete this "contract". Do not continue unless you do this!

I, _____ understand the concept of "pacing". Although not always preventable, I realize that flare-ups may be avoided if I gradually increase my activity level instead of rushing into activities.

Signature: _____

Case Study

Doctors Said He'd Never Walk Again…So Mike Learnt to Run!

In June 1989 just after midnight, Michael McGauley was tragically struck by a drunk driver and was crushed between two cars. He was rushed to the hospital but was not expected to survive the night. He remarkably survived, but after 3 days the doctors told him that they needed to amputate both his legs …but he refused! Thanks to an amazing group of surgeons, Mike received several major operations over a seven-year period, where they took a large section of muscles from his armpit to his groin and grafted it to his legs.

He had a number of complications such as infections and tissue rejections. To cope with the severe constant pain, Mike was on heavy doses of morphine and other pain medications. Doctors told him repeatedly that he would never walk again. After four years in and out of a wheelchair, Mike refused to give up. He was determined that he would not only walk again, but he would learn to run. He endured a total of 23 operations and seven long years of rehabilitation and physiotherapy.

He started training at a gym three times a week along with his daily physiotherapy sessions. Coping with severe pain, Mike slowly progressed. Finally in 1996, he permanently abandoned his wheelchair and his crutches. By June, 2001, he completed his first mini-triathlon.

What can be learned from Michael McGauley?

After being crushed between two cars, Mike was repeatedly hospitalized for nearly two years, received 23 major operations, endured several medical complications, dealt with severe pain and finally reached his physical goal. How did he do it? Here is a quote from him that will hopefully inspire you and re-assure you of your own personal recovery:

"Exercising …starting at a few to several minutes in the beginning (eventually leading) to several hours near the end -- it was not easy. It required superhuman will. But, I had firmly planted in my mind's eye the picture of myself walking around and doing things in a normal manner. That kept me going"

What is your level of hopefulness that you will improve and return to your regular activities in the next 3 months?

Not hopeful at all   Very hopeful

0   1   2   3   4   5   6   7   8   9   10

If you responded with anything less than a 9, kindly re-read Mike's story! Please don't say "…but …but, but my situation is different!"

Lesson #10: The Six Essentials of Life and Health

Oxygen: There is no question that breathing and oxygen are important to our tissue and nerve health. If you are serious about reducing your pain level, you will immediately start an appropriate exercise program that you must perform daily…yes, every single day.

This may be 5 minutes of walking three times per day, climbing two flights of stairs, cycling for three minutes or joining an aqua fitness or Tai Chi program. The goal is to get to a total of 60 minutes of moderate physical activity per day EVERY DAY!

Without adequate oxygen through a regular aerobic exercise program, your recovery is seriously delayed. It is up to you …so discuss a gentle yet progressive aerobic exercise program with your physical therapist.

Ensure that you also practice slow diaphragmatic or **abdominal breathing** several times a day (as it is done in Yoga). It is an excellent way of rejuvenating your body with oxygen.

On a final note on oxygen, do not inhale carbon monoxide …so if you smoke, see a physician to help you stop!

Do some form of aerobic exercise EVERY DAY…anything! This may be 5 minutes of walking three times per day, or joining an aqua-fitness or a Tai Chi program.

Focus on breathing only through your nose and filling your belly with air. Exhalation should last twice as long as inhalation. Breathe in through the nose for three seconds; breathe out through the nose for six seconds. Repeat several times throughout the day!

Water: Think of it, most of your body is made up of water. It seems logical that inadequate hydration can have a negative effect on tissue and nerve health. Regrettably, cups of coffee, high sugar juices, colas and beer are not considered to be the best sources of fluid. Before you panic, we are also not recommending you drink seven to ten cups of water a day.

The recommendation is eat **at least two servings of <u>fresh</u> fruits and three servings of <u>fresh</u> vegetables** each day. A slice of melon, an orange and a bowl salad are all excellent ways to hydrate your body.

The amount of water required is based on many factors including your level of physical activity. If your urine is dark yellow in colour or has a strong odour, you need to focus more on your hydration.

Do not underestimate the importance of having sufficient fluid intake. Your muscles, ligaments, discs and nerves desperately need water for health!

Food / Nutrition: Too often people have false perceptions of what a good, healthy diet is. There is so much conflicting nutritional information out there; it is next to impossible to know whom to believe. The fact is that every tissue in our body relies on the foods we consume on a daily basis to stay alive. If the nutrition, vitamins, minerals are inadequate, the tissues and nerves inevitably lose their health.

It is next to impossible to recover from a pain state without the right fuel.

It is wise to visit your family physician for a laboratory workup to see if you have any specific deficiencies such as iron, B12, vitamin D, etc. Also discuss with your physician if your muscle or joint aches may be related to side effects of excess calcium, cholesterol medications, etc.

If you experience irritable bowel syndrome or excessive bloating, you may consider visiting a registered dietician or a naturopathic doctor for a nutritional consult, to rule out specific food sensitivities such as gluten (wheat) or dairy intolerances.

Here are five sample food principles that may prove valuable in your recovery.

Avoid food products containing ingredients you:

1. Cannot pronounce *e.g. methyl cellulose, propylene glycol*
2. Cannot visualize *e.g. monosodium glutamate (MSG), Aspartame*
3. Cannot store in your pantry *e.g. high fructose corn syrup*
4. The food is likely not good for you if it arrives through your car window.
5. If the food came from a plant, it is likely good for you. If it was made in a plant, likely not!

    …Cook your own food!

Avoid foods that make health claims or that are advertised on the television.

Limit foods with a high glycemic index. There are studies that show that high blood sugar (*after eating high glycemic index foods*) immediately lowers pain thresholds and increases inflammatory reactions.

In general high glycemic index foods are:

Sugary *e.g. pastries, candy, colas, chocolate bars*
Processed *e.g. white bread, doughnuts, cake...reach for a piece of fruit instead!*

Sleep: Do you have trouble falling asleep or staying asleep? Do you get less than seven hours of sleep regularly? If yes, you need to know that many studies have clearly shown that sleep disorders can increase pain and contribute to pain.

Sleep is the most effective method the body has for resting the nervous system. As you know, **sensitized nerves** are the most common cause of persistent pain and effective deep sleep is essential for desensitizing the nervous system.

Sleep apnea is a condition where sleep is interrupted due to the inability to breathe during sleep. This condition is associated with persistent pain. Those with obesity issues, daytime sleepiness, snoring, and hypertension must be evaluated by a physician and if appropriate, referred to a sleep clinic.

If you consistently get inadequate sleep, you must speak with your health care provider. There are many drug-free suggestions for improving your sleep. Sleeping medication should be absolutely a last resort.

Studies show that just 30 minutes of walking, 4 times a week can significantly improve sleep and reduce depressive symptoms ...with no bad side effects!

The top four recommendations for improving sleep include:

1. Exercise daily to become physically tired; emotional fatigue does not help sleep.
2. Avoid tension and anxiety before bedtime. For example, no television, no newspaper, no bills, no arguments.
3. Listen to a relaxation audio program that teaches progressive physical and mental relaxation along with deep focused diaphragmatic breathing.
4. Change your old mattress, use earplugs, wear nightshades over your eyes, and if your partner snores, change rooms…(it may actually improve the relationship!).

Sun / Vitamin D: All human beings need light, sunshine and Vitamin D to survive! Several studies have shown a link between Vitamin D deficiency and chronic, 'unexplained' pain.

Amazingly, some individuals with chronic pain have shown significant improvements in their spinal pain after Vitamin D supplementation. Vitamin D insufficiency/deficiency has been reported to be common in many countries such as Canada, particularly during the winter months.

Is it not surprising that we are advised to take various painkillers and anti-inflammatory medications when all we really need is some time spent outdoors during the day in the sun?

The top three recommendations for increasing your Vitamin D levels:
1. Regularly receive midday sun exposure for 15 minutes at least twice a week exposing as much of the skin as possible. Black or brown individuals may need five times longer in the sun than those with white skin!
2. Consult your physician and if deficient, take up to 5,000 IU of Vitamin D_3/day during the winter months.
3. Eat mushrooms and vitamin D fortified beverages, such as rice milk.

Joy / Happiness: Do you know that hundreds of studies have shown that individuals with depression, anger, high stress and anxiety are at a greater risk of developing persistent pain? Do you know that job dissatisfaction has also been strongly associated with recurrence and chronicity of pain?

So what is the opposite of extreme stress, anger or anxiety? The opposite of stress, anger and anxiety is enjoying life, which unfortunately, few people who suffer from persistent pain do. As you may already know, it is not easy to be happy and joyful when you are in pain. But if there was any way of doing small things that can make you happy, smile or even laugh, it would be of tremendous physiological benefit.

Although hard to believe, just keeping a constant 'fake' smile can make a person feel better and reduce pain. Try it for one whole minute. Then try a 'fake' laugh for 15 seconds. You've got to try it…endorphins are more powerful than morphine, but without any side effects!

The top four recommendations for increasing your joy and happiness:

1. Smile for one minute, even if you have to force it!
2. Do something 'fun'…anything …walk in the park with a friend, kick a ball around for three minutes, play the piano for five minutes, go to a movie or enjoy a meal with friends, take a vacation, etc!
3. Everyday **focus on bringing joy to someone else**. Compliment others, give way in traffic, hold the door open for the person behind you, hug someone, volunteer in a hospital, seniors' home, shelter, etc.
4. Consider changing your current job or profession if you feel it is a source of unhappiness. The change may seem like an impossible task, but is your health not worth it?

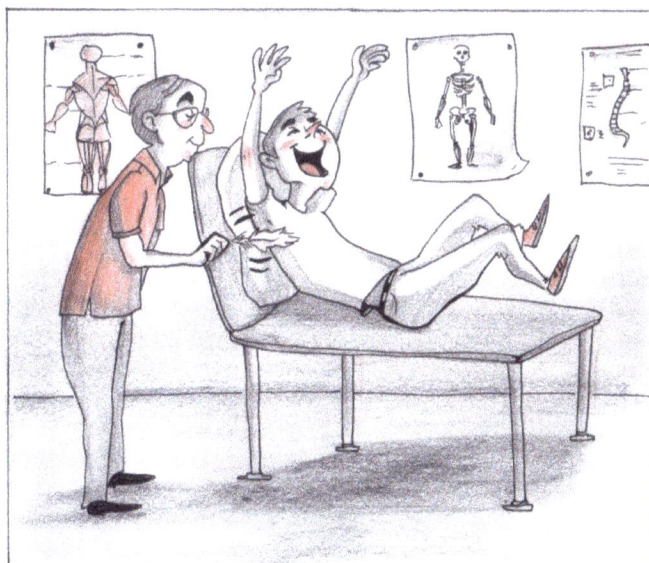

The future of helping patients in pain!

The Pain Truth Summary

Considering how complex persistent pain is, are you surprised that the management options outlined in this book have been relatively uncomplicated? Did you notice that none of the management strategies involved "purchasing" anything ...no lotions, and no fancy gadgets?

Please do not get misled by the relative simplicity of the advice provided in this book. The information is based on hundreds of medical studies published in peer-reviewed journals. The primary aim of this book was to assist those who have already seen several health care providers but continue to cope with persistent pain.

If you agree with and can **check the six boxes** that are on the next page, then follow the 16 recommendations summarized in the following pages...there is no doubt that you will see significant improvements in the quality of your life.

- ❑ You have already seen a physician who has ruled out important medical conditions such as an infection, fractures, diabetes, thyroid issues, medication side effects, etc.

- ❑ You do not currently have freshly torn muscles, ligaments or tendons (*There would be significant bleeding and black and blue bruising in the region, and a recent trauma is required.*)

- ❑ You do not currently have a pinched or compressed nerve (*There would be specific and dramatic weakness in your arms or legs e.g. a foot drop.*)

- ❑ You have already had a trial of manual therapy and possible muscle imbalances have been addressed

- ❑ If your X-ray shows "arthritis", understand that degeneration is part of a **NORMAL** aging process, and it is very rarely associated with pain

- ❑ If your MRI shows mild to moderate "disc bulges", understand that the **MAJORITY** of people with no history of pain have these "disc bulges"

The Pain Truth Summary: 16 Recommendations

1. **Understand pain** and no longer fear it, as pain does not always indicate actual damage or harm to your body.

2. Have a positive attitude; **hopefulness is a must** for recovery, not optional.

3. Set **3 goals** you wish to achieve - *e.g. Play tennis for one hour, walk in the park for 30 minutes, independently go grocery shopping.*

4. Figure out your "**easy activity**", and then gradually increase your **easy activity** by a very small amount on a daily basis.

5. **Do not panic** if you flare up, it will pass. Simply continue with progressing your easy activity.

6. Do any form of **aerobic exercise** EVERY DAY. Anything from five minutes of walking to 20 minutes of swimming …ANYTHING is good!

7. Practice slow diaphragmatic or **abdominal breathing through the nose** several times a day.

8. Drink enough **fluid**s and eat water rich foods so your urine is never dark yellow in colour with a foul odour.

9. Limit caffeinated and sugary drinks to one a day at most.

10. Do your best to prepare your own food from ingredients you can pronounce…although you can pronounce 'sugar', try to limit it!

11. Eat at least two servings of **fresh fruits** and three servings of **fresh vegetables** each day.

12. To improve your sleep, exercise daily to become **physically** tired, avoid night time stimulation, and consider listening to relaxation music.

13. Realize the value of **Vitamin D** either via the sun, foods or supplement. Get outdoors and get some light!

14. Appreciate **that high stress, depression, anger and anxiety** all influence pain. Make it your goal to deal with issues contributing to these negative emotions. You may consider seeking professional help.

15. Do something '**fun**' …anything …figure out what it is and do it ...EVERY DAY. Do not underestimate the power of smiling and **enjoying life** and helping **someone else to enjoy their life!**

16. If you feel that your current job, profession or coworkers are a source of great emotional stress and unhappiness…plan a long-term solution. Don't just sit back and hope that things will eventually change in a few years. You must be proactive, seek professional advice and make decisions.

<u>Your Participation Section</u>

Please grab a pen and paper and complete this "contract". Do not continue unless you do this!

I, _____ understand that it is very important for me to focus on the 16 recommendations above.

The three small changes I choose to start with are:

1.

2.

3.

Signature: _____

The Pain Truth Summary Sheet

✓ Pain is essential for survival; it is an alarm system that warns us of potential danger.

✓ Various medical causes of pain must be ruled out by a physician; e.g., infections, fractures, thyroid issues, diabetes, medication side effects, etc.

✓ Various mechanical causes of pain must be addressed by a physical therapist; e.g. muscle weakness, muscle tightness, joint stiffness, irritated nerves, poor posture, etc.

✓ The brain constantly evaluates all pain and determines whether to magnify or silence it.

✓ Thoughts such as fear, stress, anxiety and anger can increase pain and even produce local swelling in the painful area.

✓ 'Stress' chemicals can increase nerve hypersensitivity while 'happy' chemicals can decrease nerve hypersensitivity.

✓ **The best way to reduce the alarm sensitivity is by:**

→ Understanding pain

→ No longer fearing pain

→ Having a positive attitude

→ Setting goals

→ Pacing activities and exercises by starting with an easy activity

If you feel that you need help in finding your "**easy activity**", your goal setting and following through with your goals, I highly recommend that you consult a Pain Truth Certified (PTC) clinician.

✓ **To reduce nerve hypersensitivity, you must also address the six essentials of life and health**: **Oxygen, Water, Nutrition, Sleep, Sun, Joy & Happiness.**

If you have found the information in this book valuable, please visit www.ThePainTruth.org website and register yourself as a patient. Should you wish to continue with the 6-week Pain Truth program, you will also find a list of Pain Truth Certified (PTC) health care providers on the website. A PTC provider may be located close to you at a clinic in your area for direct consult or some offer virtual visits via video conference calling which are equally as effective.

If you have any questions, please feel free to contact me at info@thepaintruth.org

Sincerely, Bahram Jam, PT

The Pain Truth References

- Al Faraj S, Al Mutairi K. Vitamin D deficiency and chronic low back pain in Saudi Arabia. Spine. 2003 Jan 15;28(2):177-9.
- Barnard, Neal. Foods that Fight Pain. New York: Harmony Books; 1998
- Butler D & Moseley L. Explain pain. NOI Group Publications, Adelaide, Australia, 2003
- Carson JW, Keefe FJ, Lowry KP, Porter LS, Goli V, Fras AM. Conflict about expressing emotions and chronic low back pain: associations with pain and anger. J Pain. 2007 May;8(5):405-11. Epub 2007 Feb 1.
- de Roos C, Veenstra AC, de Jongh A, den Hollander-Gijsman M, van der Wee NJ, Zitman FG, van Rood YR. Treatment of chronic phantom limb pain using a trauma-focused psychological approach. Pain Res Manag. 2010 Mar-Apr;15(2):65-71.
- Doubell TP, Mannion RJ, Woolf CJ, The dorsal Horn: state dependent sensory processing, plasticity and the generation of pain, in Textbook of Pain, PD Wall and R Melzack, Editors, 1999, Churchill Livingstone: Edinburgh.
- Eccleston C, Williams AC, Morley S. Psychological therapies for the management of chronic pain (excluding headache) in adults. Cochrane Database Syst Rev. 2009 Apr 15;(2):CD007407.
- Elbert TC et al., Increased cortical representation of the fingers of the left hand in string players. Science, 1995, 270:305-307
- Fayad F, et al [Chronicity, recurrence, and return to work in low back pain: common prognostic factors] Ann Readapt Med Phys. 2004 May;47(4):179-89.
- Flor H, Braun C, Elbert T, Birbaumer N. Extensive reorganization of primary somatosensory cortex in chronic back pain patients. Neurosci Lett. 1997 Mar 7;224(1):5-8.
- Goffaux P, de Souza JB, Potvin S, Marchand S. Pain relief through expectation supersedes descending inhibitory deficits in fibromyalgia patients. Pain. 2009 Sep;145(1-2):18-23. Epub 2009 Jun 12.
- Hiestand DM, Britz P, Goldman M, Phillips B. Prevalence of symptoms and risk of sleep apnea in the US population: Results from the national sleep foundation sleep in America 2005 poll. Chest. 2006 Sep;130(3):780-6.
- Hoffman MD, Hoffman DR. Does aerobic exercise improve pain perception and mood? A review of the evidence related to healthy and chronic pain subjects. Curr Pain Headache Rep. 2007 Apr;11(2):93-7.
- Kavouras SA. Assessing hydration status. Curr Opin Clin Nutr Metab Care. 2002 Sep;5(5):519-24.
- Liu S, Manson JE, Buring JE, Stampfer MJ, Willett WC, Ridker PM. Relation between a diet with a high glycemic load and plasma concentrations of high-sensitivity C-reactive protein in middle-aged women. Am J Clin Nutr. 2002 Mar;75(3):492-8.
- Marin R, Cyhan T, Miklos W. Sleep disturbance in patients with chronic low back pain. Am J Phys Med Rehabil. 2006 May;85(5):430-5.
- Marty M, Rozenberg S, Duplan B, Thomas P, Duquesnoy B, Allaert F; Section Rachis de la Société Française de Rhumatologie. Quality of sleep in patients with chronic low back pain: a case-control study. Eur Spine J. 2008 Jun;17(6):839-44.Epub2008 Apr4.

- Morley S, Eccleston C, Williams A. Systematic review and meta-analysis of randomized controlled trials of cognitive behaviour therapy and behaviour therapy for chronic pain in adults, excluding headache. Pain. 1999 Mar;80(1-2):1-13.
- Moseley GL, Nicholas MK, Hodges PW. A randomized controlled trial of intensive neurophysiology education in chronic low back pain. Clin J Pain. 2004 Sep-Oct;20(5):324-30.
- Moseley GL. Widespread brain activity during an abdominal task markedly reduced after pain physiology education: fMRI evaluation of a single patient with chronic low back pain. Aust J Physiother. 2005;51(1):49-52.
- Moseley GL, Zalucki N, Birklein F, Marinus J, van Hilten JJ, Luomajoki H. Thinking about movement hurts: the effect of motor imagery on pain and swelling in people with chronic arm pain. Arthritis Rheum. 2008 May 15;59(5):623-31.
- Moseley GL, Brhyn L, Ilowiecki M, Solstad K, Hodges PW. The threat of predictable and unpredictable pain: differential effects on central nervous system processing? Aust J Physiother. 2003;49(4):263-7.
- Moseley GL, Nicholas MK, Hodges PW. Does anticipation of back pain predispose to back trouble? Brain. 2004 Oct;127(Pt 10):2339-47. Epub 2004 Jul 28.
- Moseley GL, Butler DS: The Explain Pain Handbook Protectometer. Noigroup publications, NOI Australasia Pty Ltd, 2015
- Pascual-Leone A, Torres F. Plasticity of the sensorimotor cortex representation of the reading finger in Braille readers. Brain. 1993 Feb;116 (Pt 1):39-52.
- Perry MC, Straker LM, Oddy WH, O'Sullivan PB, Smith AJ. Spinal pain and nutrition in adolescents - an exploratory cross-sectional study. BMC Musculoskelet Disord. 2010 Jun 30;11(1):138.
- Pincus T, Burton AK, Vogel S, Field AP. A systematic review of psychological factors as predictors of chronicity/disability in prospective cohorts of low back pain. Spine (Phila Pa 1976). 2002 Mar 1;27(5):E109-20.
- Pollan, M. Food Rules: An Eaters Manual. Penguin Books 2009
- Reid KJ, et al Aerobic exercise improves self-reported sleep and quality of life in older adults with insomnia. Sleep Med. 2010 Oct;11(9):934-40. Epub 2010 Sep 1.
- Schwalfenberg G. Improvement of chronic back pain or failed back surgery with vitamin D repletion: a case series. J Am Board Fam Med. 2009 Jan-Feb;22(1):69-74.
- Vlaeyen JW, Crombez G. Fear of movement/(re)injury, avoidance and pain disability in chronic low back pain patients. Man Ther. 1999 Nov;4(4):187-95.
- Wise TN, et al Painful physical symptoms in depression: a clinical challenge. Pain Med. 2007 Sep;8 Suppl 2:S75-82.

Advanced Physical Therapy Education Institute

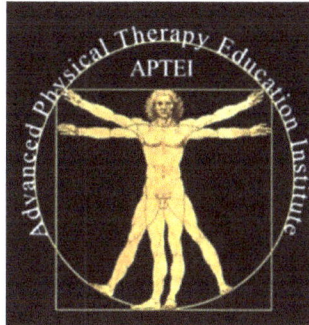

NEVER DISREGARD PROFESSIONAL MEDICAL ADVICE OR DELAY SEEKING MEDICAL TREATMENT BECAUSE OF SOMETHING YOU HAVE READ IN A BOOK OR ACCESSED THROUGH A WEBSITE.

https://www.aptei.ca

About the Author

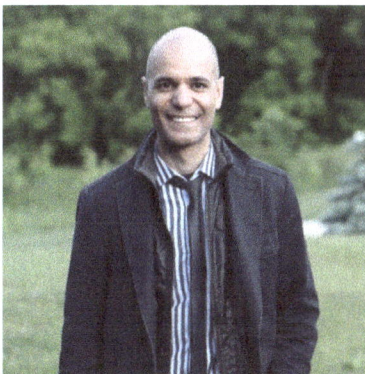

Dr. Bahram Jam graduated from the University of Toronto, Canada, in 1992 with a Bachelor of Science in Physical Therapy. In 1999 he completed a Clinical Masters in Manipulative Physiotherapy at the University of Queensland, Australia and in 2009 he completed his Doctorate of Science in Physical Therapy at Andrews University, U.S.A. He has the Canadian Diploma of Advanced Manual and Manipulative Physiotherapy and is also credentialed with the McKenzie Institute International. He is the founder and director of Advanced Physical Therapy Education Institute (APTEI) and has been a chief instructor for over one thousand post-graduate orthopedic clinical courses internationally. Bahram Jam has published several books and has presented at many national and international conferences. He continues to practice and has extensive clinical experience with direct patient care.

Understanding the Role of the Vagus Nerve in Trauma
(The Good, Bad, and What to Do About It)

Tashmeen Khimani Lalani, BA, RMT, Coach

To my amazing parents, my wonderful husband,
my incredibly supportive sister,
my beautiful daughter who is my gift from above, and
Judy, Kyle, and Justine for their unconditional love and support.

T.K.L.

Special Thanks

A special shout out to all of the survivors of trauma and their caregivers, medical professionals and educators. Warmest gratitude to my instructors, my affiliates, publicist, and publisher.

Preface

Have you ever been in so much pain and not be able to explain it? You see, everyone jumped out of the car after the motor vehicle accident but I did not immediately. I could not explain why I was so shaken up throughout the days, months, and years after. The words did not come out and the tears kept running down my face. There was something wrong and I desperately needed someone to tell me what the heck was going on with my body. I did get help, a lot of help, and hours and hours of my time learning everything about trauma. I had to change my career. I had to pivot because I love my job! Being a registered massage therapist has been my identity for over 25 years, it has been and is a part of me. I will not let that go.

I made a promise that I will keep fighting and learn everything I can so I can help myself and others to understand what is going on, how to deal with it, and what to do when they have anxiety, panic attacks and chronic physical pain. This is now my mission, and I believe, my life's purpose. I am determined. I will work hard to instruct and give a voice to the people who suffer silently and empower them. Your body is not an enemy. Your BODY MAKES SENSE. Listen to your Body, it Makes Sense. A healthy mind is a healthy body and a healthy body is a healthy mind. Please help me, help you on this healing journey from somebody who is on this journey with you.

Sincerely, Tashmeen Khimani Lalani, BA, RMT, Coach

Understanding the Role of the Vagus Nerve in Trauma

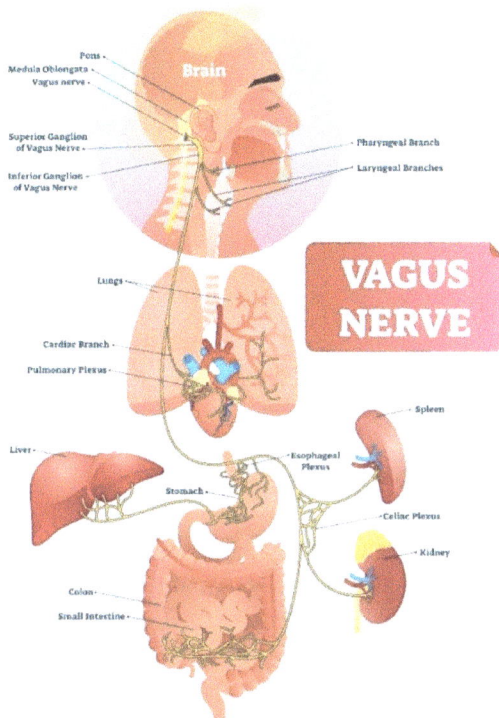

When you hear the word Vagus, what's the first thing that comes to mind? If your answer is the city in Nevada where you gamble, think again. We're talking about nerves, specifically the Cranial 10, which is more commonly referred to as the Vagus nerve. Take the advice of thousands of medical professionals; you don't want to gamble on anything when it comes to the Vagus nerve.

Before we delve into how the Vagus nerve works, we first need to have an idea of the body's nervous system and how it plays into everyday life. The brain and spinal cord make up the central nervous system. The peripheral nervous system is compromised of the somatic and autonomic nervous systems. The autonomic nervous system controls the function of our organs and glands, and can be divided into the sympathetic and parasympathetic divisions.

So, now you're probably curious about why the Vagus nerve is so important. In order to properly explain it in a relatively easy-to-understand way, let's start with the name itself. Vagus means wandering, and that's actually a good way to start describing its functions as well. Originating in the brain stem, the Vagus nerve controls the parasympathetic system in the majority of a person's internal organs. Among the organs the Vagus nerve plays a part in are the heart, the digestive tract, and even the lungs. Normally referred to in a singular form, the Vagus nerve actually has two ends, each playing an important role in your health. In the parasympathetic system alone, the Vagus can make the pupils of the eye constrict, it can slow your heartbeat, stimulate the flow of saliva, constrict your breathing passages, raises the release of bile, makes the bladder contract, and can stimulate peristalsis secretion.

To elaborate on some of the functions above, the Vagus nerve plays a crucial role in a person's health and longevity. Forming at the upper base of the spine and running all the way down to the colon, the Vagus is one of, if not the most important nerve in your body. Among its attributes is the ability to lower the heart rate, which in turn, decreases anxiety. It helps regulate insulin secretion and glucose homeostasis in the liver, which can potentially decrease the chances of diabetes. It helps the brain regulate and lower anxiety, decrease depression symptoms, and lessens the body's stress level. The Vagus nerve helps suppress inflammation; it's needed for controlling the gag reflex, swallowing, and coughing. The gut benefits by having an increase in gastric juices, which helps regulate the amount of acid in your stomach, and perhaps one of its best benefits is that it aids the blood vessels with flow and can actually lower your blood pressure!

Now that we've learned the attributes of the singular Vagus nerve, let's break it down into specifics based on the two branches. They are the Dorsal Vagus Complex and the Ventral Vagus Complex, commonly known as DVC and VVC. The DVC is the unmyelinated branch and its primary action is known as a freeze response. The VVC is a newer myelinated branch that developed in mammals and is the more social side. For the sake of example, think of a person going to a party where people they've never met will be in attendance. There are two ways a person's body will react to this event. Some people will immediately shut down and try to avoid others at all costs, while some will joyfully insert themselves into the festivities without giving it a second thought. The people who are searching for a place to hide are getting signals from the DVC branch, while the people laughing up a storm with perfect strangers are receiving signals from the VVC branch.

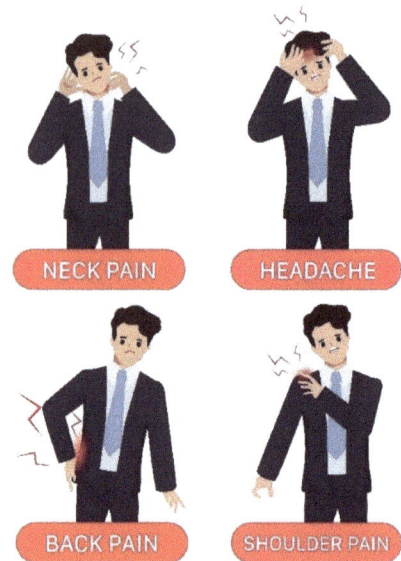

In addition to the sociologic example above, Dr. Stephen Porges developed a theory pertaining to our body's response to stresses or dangers. That theory is referred to as the Polyvagal Theory. In Dr. Porges' theory, the nervous system is broken into a three-part hierarchy based on how it activates. The first, referred to as Ventral Vagus Activation, holds the keys to relaxation and how socially engaged you are. The second is Sympathetic Activation, which controls the body's determination factor on whether to back away from something or face it head on. The third is the Dorsal Vagus Activation, which as we covered above, is the portion that creates fear and causes depression, feelings of hopelessness, and disassociates itself from others.

If a person is happy, not worrying, and essentially emotionally healthy, the body will remain in a joyous state, excited at the opportunity to be sociable with others. That's the parasympathetic activation at work. If you're constantly surrounded by stressful situations, causing your anxiety level to climb to the point of wanting to run and hide, that's the sympathetic activation. When the level of anxiety has reached a point of making you feel completely hopeless and essentially shuts down as a way of self-preservation, the unmyelinated vagus of the sympathetic nervous system has kicked in. Whether there's actually a threat to our person is irrelevant. If the body senses a perceived threat, the nervous system will do whatever it believes is necessary to protect it.

When someone experiences trauma, whether it be physical or mental, our body immediately reacts to the current circumstances. Sometimes the reaction is the desire to avenge the situation, and sometimes it's to find a quiet corner and hide until it's safe to come out. Understanding the triggers for those reactions is important so you can take steps to calm your body and ensure your mental well-being and physical safety.

How Do You Use the Vagus Nerve to Your Advantage When You Are Faced With Trauma?

Breathe: The Vagus nerve relies on stimulation to keep stress and anxiety at bay. There are simple ways to stimulate the nerve's system such as taking slow, deep breaths. Most people take 10 to 14 breaths per minute. Slowing it down to six is a great way to relieve stress. Breathe in deeply from the diaphragm and exhale slowly. Repeating this will bring your body back to a relaxing state.

Sing: Another way to stimulate the Vagus nerve is by singing. Yes, even if you're off-key and in the shower, there's nothing as refreshing as belting out your favorite songs. The Vagus nerve is attached to your vocal chords at the back of your throat, so while you're entertaining yourself and possibly others, you're also stimulating the Vagus nerve. This principle is also true of talking, humming, or anything that allows the vocal chords to move and stimulate the Vagus nerve.

Meditate: If music isn't your thing, try meditation. Meditation promotes feelings of goodwill towards yourself while stimulating the Vagus nerve and increasing the vagal tone. Breathe in through your nose while mentally counting to four. Hold your breath for two seconds, and then exhale out of your nose to the count of five or six. Repeat the method until your body relaxes itself.

Ground Yourself: Not the grounding parents used to impose that restricts your activity, but the type that reminds you that you're here, you're important, and you're safe. Stand firmly with both feet on the ground, straighten your back, relax your shoulders and slowly breathe in and out.

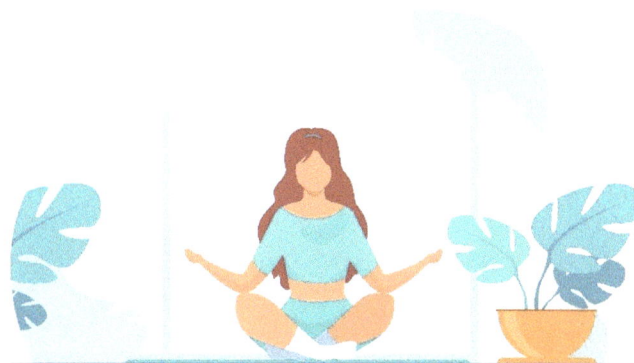

Do Something Distracting: Distract yourself with an activity. Sometimes stopping a panic attack is as simple as picking up a book or magazine, or even by baking. It's an easy premise of finding any activity that isn't focused on the cause of the anxiety or panic. When reading a book, you'll be able to focus on the words written and become absorbed in the storyline. If doing something like baking, your mind will be too focused on the recipe to continue thinking about what you're stressing about.

Identify Inner Peace with a Physical Item: Remember how Linus had his security blanket in the Peanuts™ cartoons? Your physical item doesn't necessarily have to be a blanket, but it could be a piece of jewelry, your favorite sweatshirt, anything that gives you a feeling of being secure in yourself and your surroundings. Whenever the feeling of panic begins to set in, touch the jewelry, slip into the sweatshirt if it's handy, have a cup of hot chocolate. It's usually good for conjuring good memories that will help alleviate anxious thoughts and feelings.

Get a Massage: You would be hard pressed to find anyone who doesn't appreciate a good massage, and while you're having your muscles rubbed, your Vagus nerve is lowering your stress level and evening out your vagal tone to help balance your core.

Laugh: Did you know that laughter really can be the best medicine? That's right, studies have shown that laughing and socializing with your friends can lower the stress level, increase your heart rate, and improve your mood! Research has found that reflecting on positive social interactions improves vagal tone and emotional reactions.

I'm Okay: Remind yourself that you're safe. Using both hands, touch your thumbs to the tips of each finger one at a time. As you're doing this, close your eyes and say "I am okay." Repeat this three to five times whenever it's necessary. This and the other suggestions provided will help you release the anxiety you're feeling and begin to help you let go of some of the trauma your body is healing from.

Exercise: While some us may dread going to the gym, a little exercise may be just what the doctor ordered! Mild to moderate exercise is important to maintain your body's health and it's been shown to stimulate the Vagus nerve, which increases your brain's growth hormone, supports its mitochondria, and helps reverse cognitive decline. However, and this is the important part, never make drastic changes to your diet or exercise routine without consulting your doctor first. We want to keep you healthy inside and out.

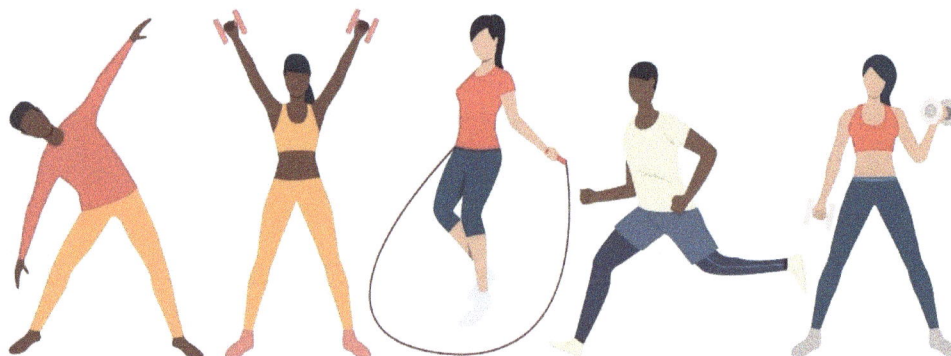

Aromatherapy: Another great way to almost instantly relax is with aromatherapy. Have you ever noticed how quickly the scent of lavender helps you relax? It's because it increases your heart rate variability and improves vagal tone.

Yoga: This leads us to Yoga. Are you aware that the activation of the Vagus nerve helps keep your immune system healthy and releases an assortment of hormones that can help reduce inflammation, reduce allergy symptoms, offer relief from tension headaches, as well as improve memory functions, and supply feelings of relaxation? The Vagus nerve passes through the belly, diaphragm, lungs, throat, inner ear, and facial muscle. In fact, 80% of the vagus nerve fibers are sensory nerves, meaning they communicate messages from your body back up to your central nervous system. When you move and breathe into these areas of the body, you're influencing the function of your Vagus nerve.

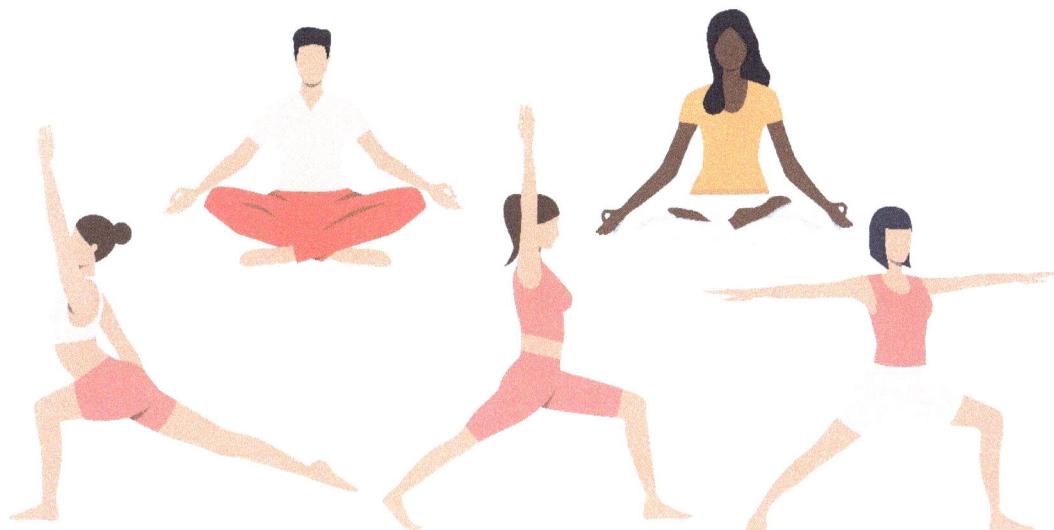

Natural Vagus stimulation explores gentle yoga breathing and movements that aim to stimulate and balance the Vagus nerve. Slowing down how you exhale is considered one of the most direct ways to balance the nerve. Emphasis on emptying the lungs through the diaphragm and abdominal muscles not only stimulates the nerve fibers in the lungs, but provides a gentle massage to the digestive organs.

So let's talk about digestion. When you digest food, the Vagus nerve sends a signal to your brain. For example, let's say you're sensitive to a certain spice. Not necessarily allergic to it, but it's still enough to cause digestive discomfort. The stomach or intestinal area sends a message through the Vagus nerve to your brain to let you know that the irritation is happening. Your brain sends a message back through the Vagus nerve that initiates the process to reduce the potential intestinal inflammation taking place. When the Vagus nerve isn't stimulated, it can't send the necessary messages and signals to stop your body from sustaining damage. That not only contributes to the assorted digestive disorders above, but can also affect your heart, liver, kidneys, and even your tongue. Being part of the parasympathetic nervous system, it's not only responsible for digestion, but emotional well-being. Take this information as food for thought and remember to always think about the food you're putting into your body.

Irregularity in the Vagus nerve is a cause of distress in a person's overall physical and mental health. Physical issues that can appear include gastroesophageal reflux disease (GERD or severe Acid Reflux), irritable bowel syndrome (IBS), nausea, vomiting, fainting, tinnitus, autoimmune disorders, migraines, and seizures. Mental health issues can include fatigue, depression, and anxiety, overwhelming feelings, wanting to mentally shut down, and panic attacks.

Let's get to work on some of the techniques that may help you.

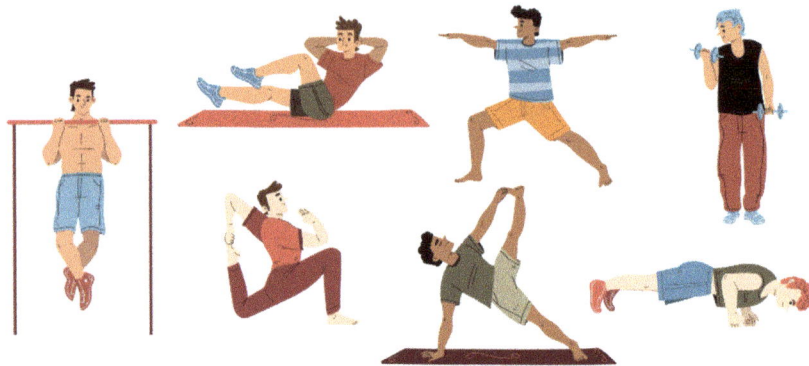

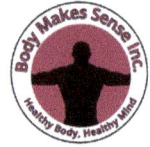

BODY MAKES SENSE INC.

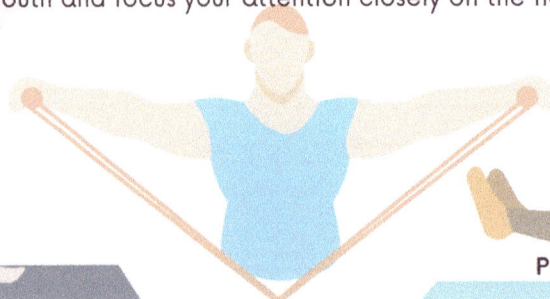

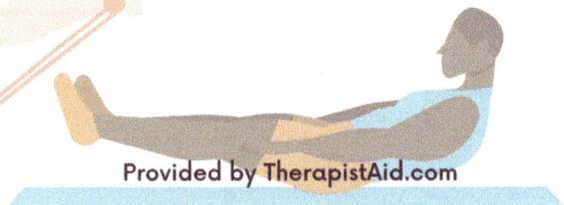

GROUNDING TECHNIQUES

After a trauma, it's normal to experience flashbacks, anxiety, and other uncomfortable symptoms. **Grounding techniques** help control these symptoms by turning attention away from thoughts, memories, or worries, and refocusing on the present moment.

5-4-3-2-1 Technique

Using the 5-4-3-2-1 technique, you will purposefully take in the details of your surroundings using each of your senses. Strive to notice small details that your mind would usually tune out, such as distant sounds, or the texture of an ordinary object.

What are 5 things you can see? Look for small details such as a pattern on the ceiling, the way light reflects off a surface, or an object you never noticed.

What are 4 things you can feel? Notice the sensation of clothing on your body, the sun on your skin, or the feeling of the chair you are sitting in. Pick up an object and examine its weight, texture, and other physical qualities.

What are 3 things you can hear? Pay special attention to the sounds your mind has tuned out, such as a ticking clock, distant traffic, or trees blowing in the wind.

What are 2 things you can smell? Try to notice smells in the air around you, like an air freshener or freshly mowed grass. You may also look around for something that has a scent, such as a flower or an unlit candle.

What is 1 thing you can taste? Carry gum, candy, or small snacks for this step. Pop one in your mouth and focus your attention closely on the flavors.

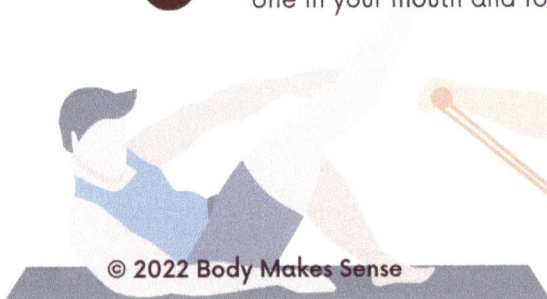

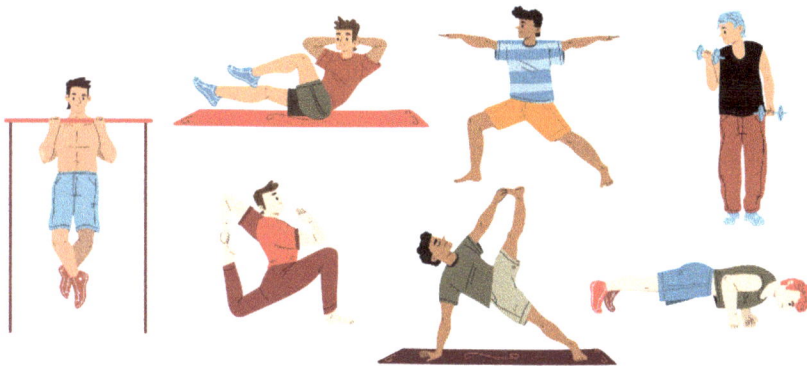

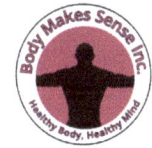

BODY MAKES SENSE INC.

Categories

Choose at least three of the categories below and name as many items as you can in each one. Spend a few minutes on each category to come up with as many items as possible.

Movies	Countries	Books	Cereals
Sport Teams	Colors	Cars	Fruits & Vegetables
Animals	Cities	TV Shows	Famous People

For a variation on this activity, try naming items in a category alphabetically. For example, for the fruits & vegetables category, say "apple, banana, carrot," and so on.

Body Awareness

The body awareness technique will bring you into the here-and-now by directing your focus to sensations in the body. Pay special attention to the physical sensations created by each step.

1. Take 5 long, deep breaths through your nose, and exhale through puckered lips.
2. Place both feet flat on the floor. Wiggle your toes. Curl and uncurl your toes several times. Spend a moment noticing the sensations in your feet.
3. Stomp your feet on the ground several times. Pay attention to the sensations in your feet and legs as you make contact with the ground.
4. Clench your hands into fists, then release the tension. Repeat this 10 times.
5. Press your palms together. Press them harder and hold this pose for 15 seconds. Pay attention to the feeling of tension in your hands and arms.
6. Rub your palms together briskly. Notice and sound and the feeling of warmth.
7. Reach your hands over your head like you're trying to reach the sky. Stretch like this for 5 seconds. Bring your arms down and let them relax at your sides.
8. Take 5 more deep breaths and notice the feeling of calm in your body.

Provided by TherapistAid.com

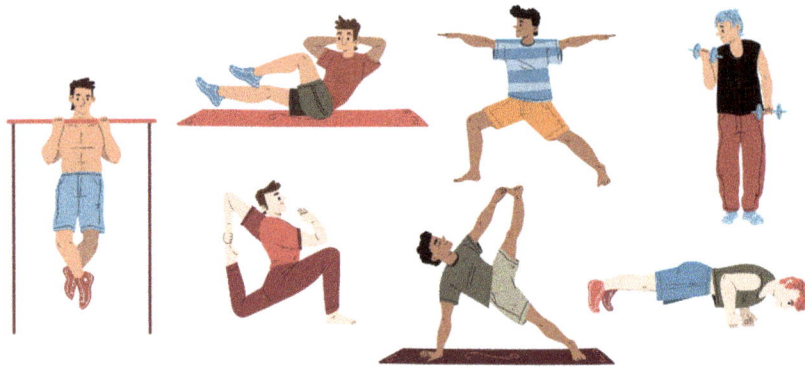

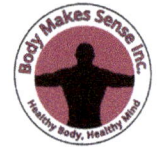

BODY MAKES SENSE INC.

Mental Exercises

Use mental exercises to take your mind off uncomfortable thoughts and feelings. They are discreet and easy to use at nearly any time or place. Experiment to see which work best for you.

- Name all the objects you see.
- Describe the steps in performing an activity you know how to do well. For example, how to shoot a basketball, prepare your favorite meal, or tie a knot.
- Count backwards from 100 by 7.
- Pick up an object and describe it in detail. Describe its color, texture, size, weight, scent, and any other qualities you notice.
- Spell your full name, and the names of three other people, backwards.
- Name all your family members, their ages, and one of their favorite activities.
- Read something backwards, letter-by-letter. Practice for at least a few minutes.
- Think of an object and "draw" it in your mind, or in the air with your finger. Try drawing your home, a vehicle, or an animal.

References:
1. Najavits, L. (2002). Seeking safety: A treatment manual for PTSD and substance abuse. Guilford Publications.

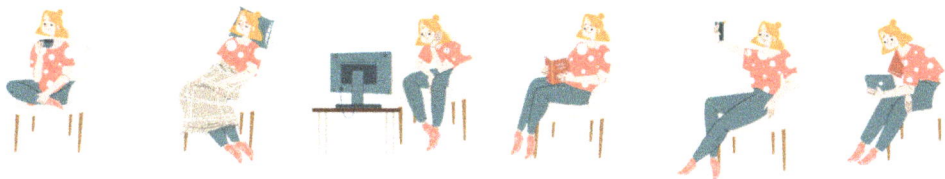

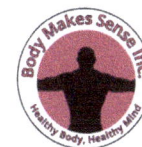

BODY MAKES SENSE INC.

RELAXATION TECHNIQUES

When a person is confronted with anxiety, their body undergoes several changes and enters a special state called the fight-or-flight response. The body prepares to either fight or flee the perceived danger.

During the fight-or-flight response it's common to experience a "blank" mind, increased heart rate, sweating, tense muscles, and more. Unfortunately, these bodily responses do little good when it comes to protecting us from modern sources of anxiety.

Using a variety of skills, you can end the fight-or-flight response before the symptoms become too extreme. These skills will require practice to work effectively, so don't wait until the last minute to try them out!

Deep Breathing

It's natural to take long, deep breaths, when relaxed. However, during the fight-or-flight response, breathing becomes rapid and shallow. Deep breathing reverses that, and sends messages to the brain to begin calming the body. Practice will make your body respond more efficiently to deep breathing in the future.

1. Breathe in slowly. Count in your head and make sure the inward breath lasts at least 5 seconds. Pay attention to the feeling of the air filling your lungs.
2. Hold your breath for 5 to 10 seconds (again, keep count). You don't want to feel uncomfortable, but it should last quite a bit longer than an ordinary breath.
3. Breathe out very slowly for 5 to 10 seconds (count!). Pretend like you're breathing through a straw to slow yourself down. Try using a real straw to practice.
4. Repeat the breathing process until you feel calm.

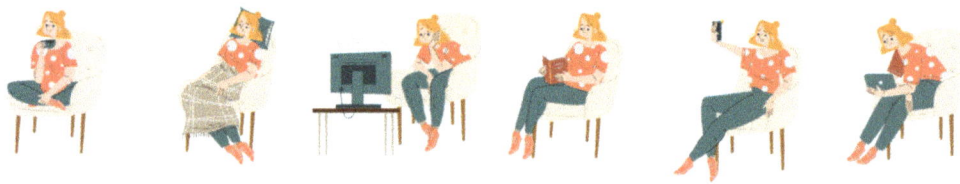

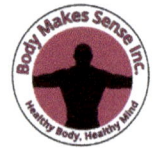

BODY MAKES SENSE INC.

Imagery

Think about some of your favorite and least favorite places. If you think about the place hard enough—if you really try to think about what it's like—you may begin to have feelings you associate with that location. Our brain has the ability to create emotional reactions based entirely off of our thoughts. The imagery technique uses this to its advantage.

1. Make sure you're somewhere quiet without too much noise or distraction. You'll need a few minutes to just spend quietly, in your mind.

2. Think of a place that's calming for you. Some examples are the beach, hiking on a mountain, relaxing at home with a friend, or playing with a pet.

3. Paint a picture of the calming place in your mind. Don't just think of the place briefly—imagine every little detail. Go through each of your senses and imagine what you would experience in your relaxing place. Here's an example using a beach:

   a. Sight: The sun is high in the sky and you're surrounded by white sand. There's no one else around. The water is a greenish-blue and waves are calmly rolling in from the ocean.

   b. Sound: You can hear the deep pounding and splashing of the waves. There are seagulls somewhere in the background.

   c. Touch: The sun is warm on your back, but a breeze cools you down just enough. You can feel sand moving between your toes.

   d. Taste: You have a glass of lemonade that's sweet, tart, and refreshing.

   e. Smell: You can smell the fresh ocean air, full of salt and calming aromas.

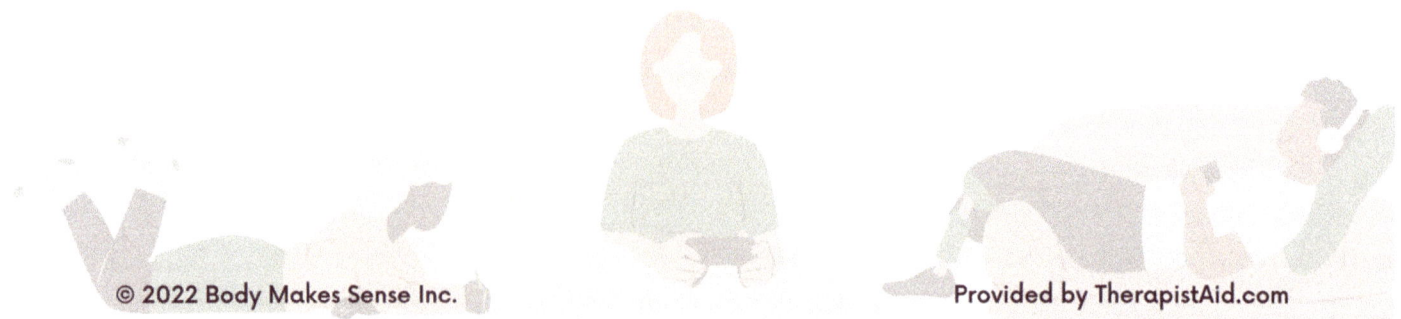

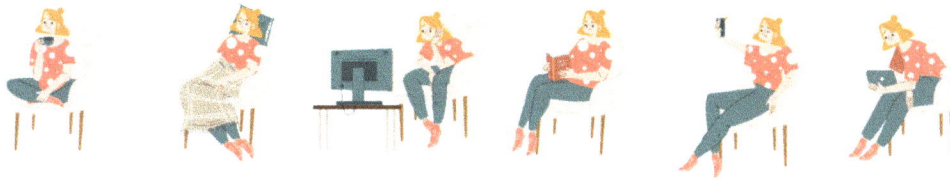

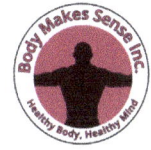

BODY MAKES SENSE INC.

Progressive Muscle Relaxation

During the fight-or-flight response, the tension in our muscles increases. This can lead to a feeling of stiffness, or even back and neck pain. Progressive muscle relaxation teaches us to become more aware of this tension so we can better identify and address stress.

Find a private and quiet location. You should sit or lie down somewhere comfortable.

The idea of this technique is to intentionally tense each muscle, and then to release the tension. Let's practice with your feet.

- Tense the muscles in your toes by curling them into your foot. Notice how it feels when your foot is tense. Hold the tension for 5 seconds.
- Release the tension from your toes. Let them relax. Notice how your toes feel differently after you release the tension.
- Tense the muscles all throughout your calf. Hold it for 5 seconds. Notice how the feeling of tension in your leg feels.
- Release the tension from your calf, and notice how the feeling of relaxation differs.

Follow this pattern of tensing and releasing tension all throughout your body. After you finish with your feet and legs, move up through your torso, arms, hands, neck, and head.

References:
1. Apóstolo, J. L. A., & Kolcaba, K. (2009). The effects of guided imagery on comfort, depression, anxiety, and stress of psychiatric inpatients with depressive disorders. Archives of psychiatric nursing, 23(6), 403-411.
2. Hazlett-Stevens, H., & Craske, M. G. (2009). Breathing retraining and diaphragmatic breathing. General principles and empirically supported techniques of cognitive behavior therapy.
3. McCallie, M. S., Blum, C. M., & Hood, C. J. (2006). Progressive muscle relaxation. Journal of Human Behavior in the Social Environment, 13(3), 51-66.

Provided by TherapistAid.com

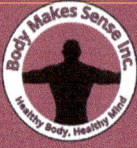

BODY MAKES SENSE INC.
GRATITUDE EXERCISES

Gratitude means appreciating the good things in life, no matter how big or small. Making the practice of gratitude a regular part of your day can build happiness, self-esteem, and provide other health benefits.

Gratitude Journal

Every evening, spend a few minutes writing down some good things about your day. This isn't limited to major events. You might be grateful for simple things, such as a good meal, talking to a friend, or overcoming an obstacle.

Give Thanks

Keep your eyes open throughout the day for reasons to say "thank you." Make a conscious effort to notice when people do good things, whether for you or others. Tell the person you recognize their good deed, and give a sincere "thank you."

Mindfulness Walk

Go for a walk and make a special effort to appreciate your surroundings. You can do this by focusing on each of your senses, one at a time. Spend a minute just listening, a minute looking at your surroundings, and so on. Try to notice the sights, sounds, smells, and sensations you would usually miss, such as a cool breeze on your skin, or the clouds in the sky.

Provided by TherapistAid.com

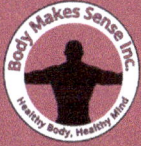

BODY MAKES SENSE INC.
GRATITUDE EXERCISES

Gratitude Letter

Think about someone who you appreciate. This could be a person who has had a major impact on your life, or someone who you would like to thank. Write a letter that describes why you appreciate them, including specific examples and details. It's up to you if you'd like to share the letter or not.

Grateful Contemplation

Remove yourself from distractions such as phones or TV and spend 5-10 minutes mentally reviewing the good things from your day. The key to this technique is consistency. Think of it like brushing your teeth or exercise—it should be a normal part of daily self-care. This technique can be practiced as part of prayer, meditation, or on its own.

Gratitude Conversation

With another person, take turns listing 3 things you were grateful for throughout the day. Spend a moment discussing and contemplating each point, rather than hurrying through the list. Make this part of your routine by practicing before a meal, before bed, or at another regular time.

References:
1. Lambert, N. M., Graham, S. M., & Fincham, F. D. (2009). A prototype analysis of gratitude: Varieties of gratitude experiences. Personality and Social Psychology Bulletin, 35(9), 1193-1207.
2. Rash, J. A., Matsuba, M. K., & Prkachin, K. M. (2011). Gratitude and well-being: Who benefits the most from a gratitude intervention?. Applied Psychology: Health and Well-Being, 3(3), 350-369.
3. Watkins, P. C., Emmons, R. A., & McCullough, M. E. (2004). Gratitude and subjective well-being.
4. Wilson, J. T. (2016). Brightening the mind: The impact of practicing gratitude on focus and resilience in learning. Journal of the Scholarship of Teaching and Learning, 16(4), 1-13.
5. Wood, A. M., Froh, J. J., & Geraghty, A. W. (2010). Gratitude and well-being: A review and theoretical integration. Clinical psychology review, 30(7), 890-905.

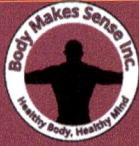

BODY MAKES SENSE INC.
GRATITUDE JOURNAL

Day 1

One good thing that happened to me today...

Something good that I saw someone do...

Today I had fun when...

Day 2

Something I accomplished today...

Something funny that happened today...

Provided by TherapistAid.com

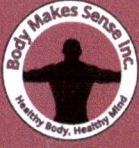

BODY MAKES SENSE INC.
GRATITUDE JOURNAL

Someone I was thankful for today...

Day 3

Something I was thankful for today...

Today I smiled when...

Something about today I'll always want to remember...

Day 4

One good thing that happened to me today...

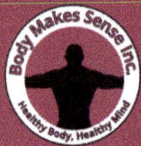

BODY MAKES SENSE INC.
GRATITUDE JOURNAL

Today was special because...

Today I was proud of myself because...

Day 5

Something interesting that happened today...

Someone I was thankful for today...

Today I had fun when...

Provided by TherapistAid.com

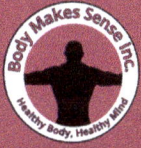

BODY MAKES SENSE INC.
GRATITUDE JOURNAL

Day 6

Something about today I'll always want to remember...

Something funny that happened today...

My favorite part of today...

Day 7

Something I was happy about today...

Something good I saw someone do today...

Provided by TherapistAid.com

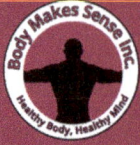

BODY MAKES SENSE INC.
GRATITUDE JOURNAL

Something I did well today...

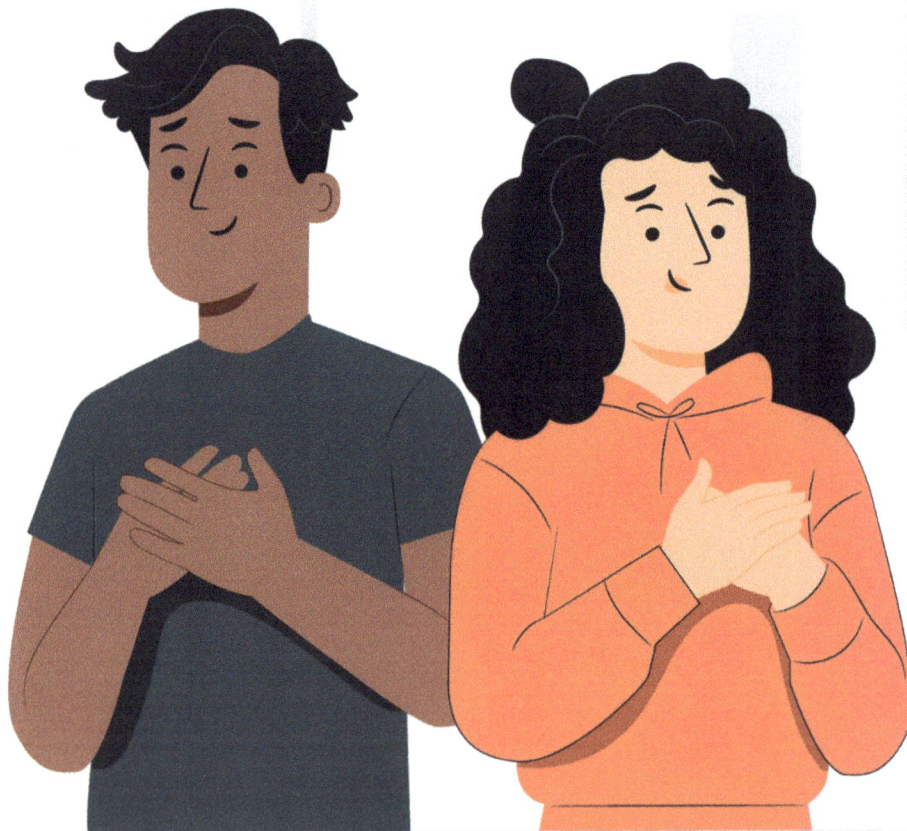

Provided by TherapistAid.com

Pain Truth Makes Sense Summary

When you feel safe and at peace, living in a harmonious state, your parasympathetic nervous system offers an energetic sigh of relief that flows throughout your entire being as a fusion of calm, clarity, compassion, and connectedness that positively fuels your body systems. It's at the heart of radiant health and a beautiful life. The Pain Truth and Understanding the role of the Vagus Nerve restores balance within your body systems, increases circulation, and boosts your immunity and vibration... heightening your own body's innate ability to self-heal. When you establish a higher baseline, **EVERY** part of your life benefits.

Thank you for letting us be a part of your healing journey.

Listen to your Body, it Makes Sense.

Body Makes Sense Inc.

A Healthy Mind is a Healthy Body, A Healthy Body is a Healthy Mind.

Visit our website!
www.bodymakessense.com/

~ Incredible Bonus Experience ~
https://bit.ly/3Pfp42J

Join our Movement on Facebook and Instagram!

Understanding the Role of the Vagus Nerve in Trauma References

- Apóstolo, J. L. A., & Kolcaba, K. (2009). The effects of guided imagery on comfort, depression, anxiety, and stress of psychiatric inpatients with depressive disorders. Archives of psychiatric nursing, 23(6), 403-411.
- Begley, S. and Davidson, R. (2013). The Emotional Life of Your Brain: How Its Unique Patterns Affect the Way You Think, Feel and Live - and How You Can Change Them. Hodder Paperbacks.
- Benson, H. (1975). The Relaxation Response. New York: Morrow.
- Burrell, L. (2019). EMF Practical Guide: The Simple Science of protecting Yourself, Healing Chronic Inflammation, and Living a Naturally Healthy Life in our Toxic Electromagnetic World. AFNIL.
- Crum, A. J. and Langer, E. J. (2007). Mind-Set Matters: Exercise and the Placebo Effect, Psychol Sci; vol. 18, no. 2: pp. 165-171.
- Dana, D. (2020). Polyvagal Exercises for Safety and Connection. 50 Client-Centered Practices (Norton Series on Interpersonal Neurobiology). W. W. Norton & Company.
- Davidson, R. J., Jackson, D. C. and Kalin, N. H. (2000). Emotion, Plasticity, Context, and Regulation: Perspectives from Affective Neuroscience. Psychol Bulletin, 126(6), 890.
- Detko, E. (2022). The Sovereign Health Method: Addressing the Psycho-Energetic Root Causes of Chronic Illness. Lifestyle Entrepreneurs Press.
- Dillon, K. M., Minchoff, B. and Baker, K. H. (1985-1986) Positive Emotional States and Enhancement of the Immune System. Int J Psych Med; vol. 15, no. 1: pp. 13-18.
- Dispenza, J. (2012). Breaking the Habit of Being Yourself: How to Lose Your Mind and Create a New One. Hay House UK.
- Dispenza, J. (2014). You Are the Placebo: Making Your Mind Matter, Hay House UK.
- Fehmiand L. and Robbins J. (2007). The Open-Focus Brain: Harnessing the Power of Attention to Heal Mind and Body. Boston: Trumpeter Books.
- Gratitude Exercises. (n.d.). Therapist Aid. Retrieved August 9, 2022, from https://www.therapistaid.com/therapy-worksheet/gratitude-exercises
- Grounding Techniques. (n.d.). Therapist Aid. Retrieved August 9, 2022, from https://www.therapistaid.com/therapy-worksheet/grounding-techniques
- Habib, N. (2019). Activate Your Vagus Nerve: Unleash Your Body's Natural Ability to Heal. Ulysses Press; Illustrated edition.
- Hamilton, D. R. (2010). How Your Mind Can Heal Your Body. Carlsbad, CA: Hay House.
- Harris, T. A. (1973). I'm OK - You're OK. Pan Books Ltd.
- Hay. L. (1984). You Can Heal Your Life Hay House; New edition.
- Hazlett-Stevens, H., & Craske, M. G. (2009). Breathing retraining and diaphragmatic breathing. General principles and empirically supported techniques of cognitive behavior therapy.
- Heim, C. and Nemeroff, C. B. (2009). Neurobiology of Posttraumatic Stress Disorder. CNS spectr, 14(1 suppl. 1), 13-24.

- Jacobs Hendel, H. (2018). It's Not Always Depression: Working the Change Triangle to Listen to the Body, Discover Core Emotions, and Connect to Your Authentic Self. Penguin Life.
- Kok, B. E. et al. (2013). How Positive Emotions Build Physical Health: Perceived Positive Social Connections Account for the Upward Spiral Between Positive Emotions and Vagal Tone. Psychol Sci; vol. 24, no. 7:pp. 1123-1132.
- Lambert, N. M., Graham, S. M., & Fincham, F. D. (2009). A prototype analysis of gratitude: Varieties of gratitude experiences. Personality and Social Psychology Bulletin, 35(9), 1193-1207.
- Levine, A. and Heller, R. (2019). Attached: Are you Anxious, Avoidant or Secure? How the science of adult attachment can help you find and keep love Bluebird; Main Market edition.
- Levine, P. (1997). Waking The Tiger: Healing Trauma. North Atlantic Books, Berkeley CA.
- Lipton, B. (2005). The Biology of Belief. Unleashing the Power of Consciousness, Matter & Miracles. Hay House Inc.
- McCallie, M. S., Blum, C. M., & Hood, C. J. (2006). Progressive muscle relaxation. Journal of Human Behavior in the Social Environment, 13(3), 51-66.
- Myss, C. (1998). Why People Don't Heal And How They Can: a guide to healing and overcoming physical and mental illness. Bantam; 1st Paperback.
- Najavits, L. (2002). Seeking safety: A treatment manual for PTSD and substance abuse. Guilford Publications.
- Newbigging, S. C. (2019) Mind Detox: Discover and Resolve the Root Causes of Chronic Conditions and Persistent Problems. Findhorn Press; 2nd edition.
- Oschman, J. L. (2006). Trauma Energetics. J Bodyw Mov Ther; vol 10 no. 1: pp. 21-34.
- Pert, C.B. (1997). Molecules of Emotion. Why You Feel the Way You Feel. Scribner, New York.
- Pitman, R. K. (1989). Post-traumatic Stress Disorder, Hormones, and Memory. Biol Psych; 26(3), 221-223.
- Porges, S. W (2021). Polyvagal Safety: Attachment, Communication, Self-Regulation. WW Norton & Co.
- Ranganathan, V. K et al. (2004). From Mental Power to Muscle Power: Gaining Strength by Using the Mind. Neuropsychologia; vol. 42, no. 7: pp. 944-956.
- Rankin, L. (2020). Mind Over Medicine: Scientific Proof That You Can Heal Yourself Hay House Inc; revised edition.
- Rash, J. A., Matsuba, M. K., & Prkachin, K. M. (2011). Gratitude and well-being: Who benefits the most from a gratitude intervention? Applied Psychology: Health and Well-Being, 3(3), 350-369.
- Relaxation Techniques. (n.d.). Therapist Aid. Retrieved August 9, 2022, from https://www.therapistaid.com/therapy-worksheet/relaxation-techniques
- Rosenzweig, M. R. and Bennett, E. L. (1996). Psychobiology of Plasticity: Effects of Training and Experience on Brain and Behavior. Behav Brain Res; vol. 78, no. 1: pp. 57-65.
- Rusk, T. and Read, R. (1986). I Want to Change But I Don't Know How. Price/Stern/Sloan Publishers, Inc., Los Angeles.
- Sareen, J. (2014). Posttraumatic Stress Disorder in Adults; Impact, Comorbidity, Risk Factors, and Treatment. Can J Psych; 59(9), 460-467.

- Schauer, M. and Elbert, T. (2010). Dissociation Following Traumatic Stress: Etiology and Treatment. J Psychol; 218(2), 109-127.

- Sherin, J. E. and Nemeroff, C. B. (2011). Post-traumatic Stress Disorder: the Neurobiological Impact of Psychological Trauma. Dial Clin Neurosci; 13(3), 263.

- Tugade, M. M. and Fredrickson, B. L. (2004). Resilient Individuals Use Positive Emotions to Bounce Back from Negative Emotional Experiences. J Pers Soc Psycho; Feb: 86(2):320-33.

- Tugade, M. M. et al. (2004). Psychological Resilience and Positive Emotional Granularity: Examining the Benefits of Positive Emotions on Coping and Health.i pets; Dec: 72(6):1161-90.

- Van der Kolk, B.A. (2014). The Body Keeps the Score: Mind, Brain and Body in the Transformation of Trauma. Penguin; 1st edition.

- Watkins, P. C., Emmons, R. A., & McCullough, M. E. (2004). Gratitude and subjective well-being.

- Wilson, J. T. (2016). Brightening the mind: The impact of practicing gratitude on focus and resilience in learning. Journal of the Scholarship of Teaching and Learning, 16(4), 1-13.

- Wood, A. M., Froh, J. J., & Geraghty, A. W. (2010). Gratitude and well-being: A review and theoretical integration. Clinical psychology review, 30(7), 890-905.

About the Author

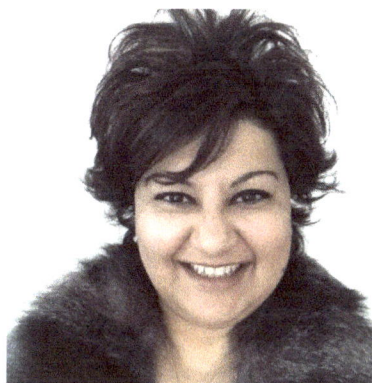

Tashmeen Khimani Lalani is a Registered Massage Therapist with Natural Health Practitioners of Canada and has over 25 years of experience of giving massages in all clinical settings. She has a Bachelor of Arts degree with a double major in Psychology and Linguistics. She is a Life Coach, Health Coach, Wellness Coach and Body Healing Coach. She is a Yin Yoga Instructor and is well rehearsed in Trauma Informed Yoga and Anxiety. She has completed several training and certificates in Mental Health First Aid Canada, Somatic Approaches to Healing Trauma, Integrative Somatic Trauma Therapy. Advanced Master program on the Treatment of Trauma and that is just to name a few. Tashmeen is now on the Biology of Trauma Network. She is continually growing and reaching for the stars.

Body Makes Sense:
Listen to Your Body, It Makes Sense

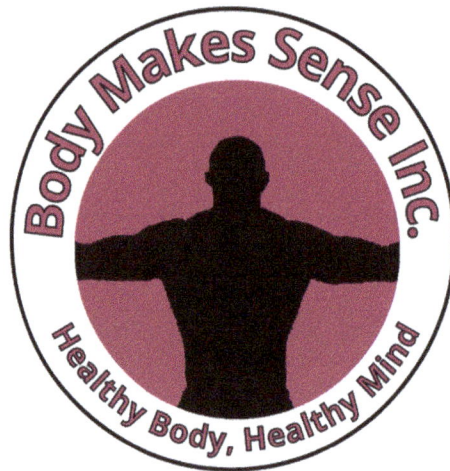

NEVER DISREGARD PROFESSIONAL MEDICAL ADVICE OR DELAY SEEKING MEDICAL TREATMENT BECAUSE OF SOMETHING YOU HAVE READ IN A BOOK OR ACCESSED THROUGH A WEBSITE.

Visit our website!
www.bodymakessense.com/

~ Incredible Bonus Experience ~
https://bit.ly/3Pfp42J

Join our Movement on Facebook and Instagram!

www.ingramcontent.com/pod-product-compliance
Lightning Source LLC
Chambersburg PA
CBHW042347030426
42335CB00031B/3485